ADVICE AND RECIPES BY EXPERTS

Eating Guide for Fussy Kids

Eirini Togia
Chef and Author

Pavlos Sakkas
Professor of Psychiatry,
National and Kapodistrian University of Athens

George Moustakas
Paediatrician

Stergiou Limited
United Kingdom
2018

COPYRIGHT
© 2018 by Eirini Togia

CATALOGUING IN PUBLICATION DATA
British Library

PUBLISHER
Stergiou Limited
Suite A, 6 Honduras St., London EC1Y 0TH, United Kingdom
publications@stergioultd.com | stergioubooks.com

AUTHOR
Eirini Togia ("Rena tis Ftelias")

MEDICAL ADVISORS — CO AUTHORS
Pavlos Sakkas, George Moustakas

TITLE
Eating Guide for Fussy Eaters: Advice and Recipes by Experts

ENGLISH EDITION
Paperback ISBN (Primary): 978-1-912315-36-9
Paperback ISBN (Amazon edition): 978-1-912315-18-5
Ebook (standard edition) ISBN: 978-1-912315-19-2
Ebook (fixed-layout/print replica) ISBN: 978-1-912315-35-2

ORIGINAL EDITION - GREEK LANGUAGE (MARCH 2018)
Paperback ISBN: 978-1-912315-16-1
Ebook ISBN: 978-1-912315-17-8

EDITOR
Leonidas Stergiou

TRANSLATOR AND COPY-EDITOR
Catherine Pavlou Evans

COVER ILLUSTRATOR
© Doloves | iStock.com
INTERIOR DESIGN
© Themzy | stock.adobe.com. Adaptation: Stergiou Limited

PHOTOS
Vangelis Paterakis, Efstratios Havaletzis, Leonidas Stergiou,
Adobe Stock, Burst, iStock, Pexel, Pixabay

PERMISSIONS
NHS.UK Choices | www.nhs.uk

Dedication

To all children and parents.

Contents

Section 1
Advice from the experts.

Causes and common mistakes members of the family make and practical advice to solve them.

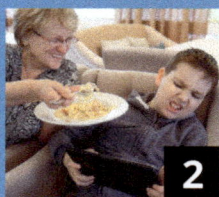

2

Section 2
Delicacies by Chef Eirini Togia.

The goal: make children love eating.

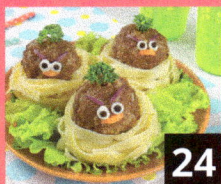

24

Contents

Section 3
Dad shares his own experience.

From Chef Eirini Togia he gathered inspiration; the imagination, the dishes, and the tricks are all his.

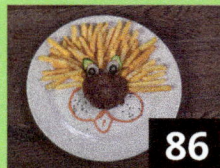

86

Section 4
A true story.

The torture of eating and the psy-chiatrist's comment.

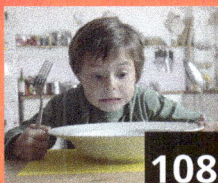

108

Section 5
Guide.

Expert tips.

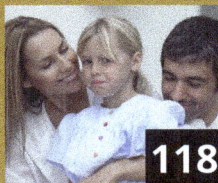

118

Contents

Figures

Picky eaters in the United States

Which of the following people, if any, do you consider to be picky eaters?

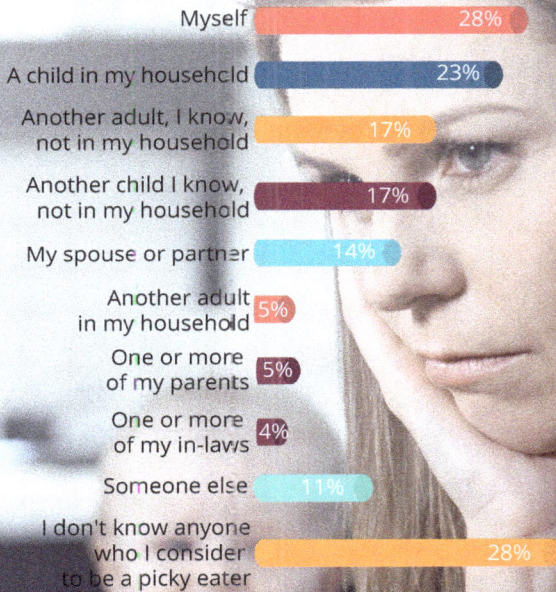

Category	Percentage
Myself	28%
A child in my household	23%
Another adult, I know, not in my household	17%
Another child I know, not in my household	17%
My spouse or partner	14%
Another adult in my household	5%
One or more of my parents	5%
One or more of my in-laws	4%
Someone else	11%
I don't know anyone who I consider to be a picky eater	28%

2,232 respondents; 18 years and older, USA, 2015. Multiple responses were possible.

Figure 1: Harris Interactive
© Statista 2018

© highwaystarz | stock.adobe.com

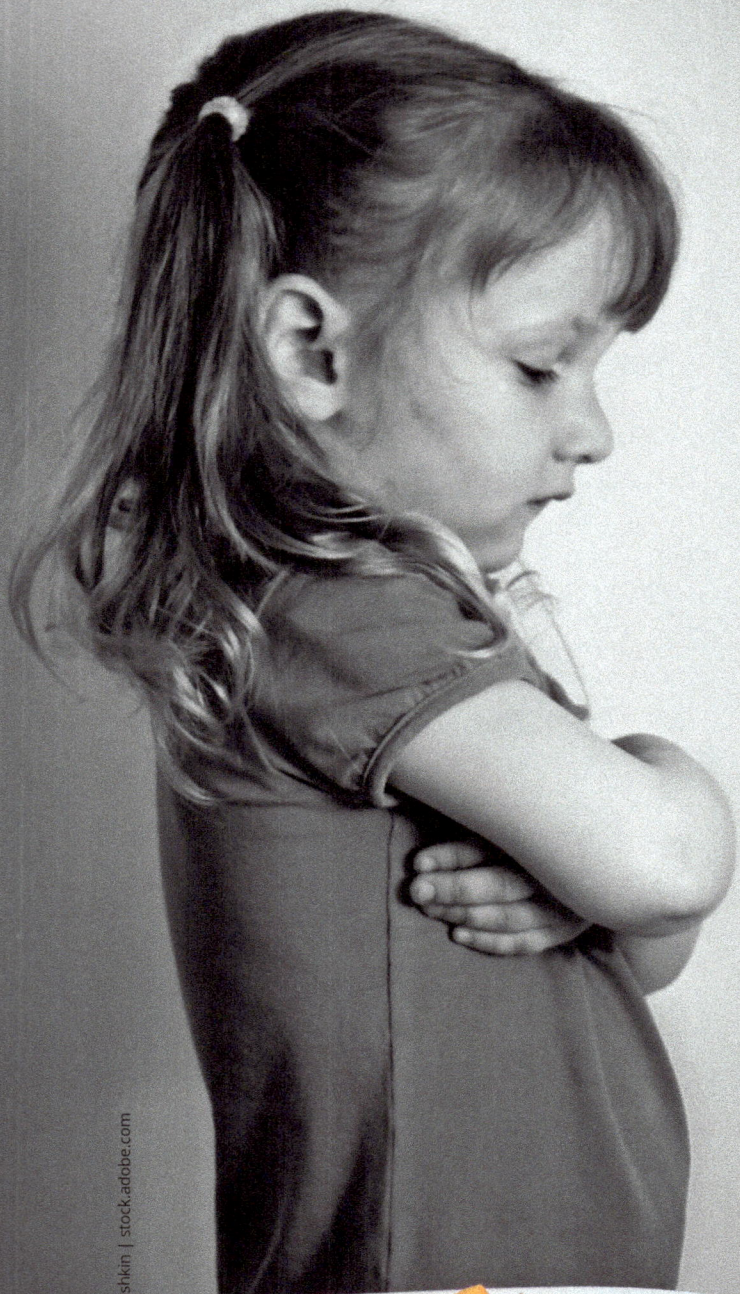

Editor's preface

It is not by coincidence that the authors and the editor of this book are all of Mediterranean origin. In this part of the world, food is a severe issue! The same applies to the family. And they are best expressed together on the occasion of a joyful family feast.

So, in the Mediterranean culture, a picky or fuzzy eater is a matter of concern that is worthy of attention. A holistic approach was the concept of the first edition, published earlier this year in Greece. It aimed to help expand a child's appetite as well as to highlight the family dynamics that may trigger this kind of behaviour.

The success of the first Greek edition as well as substantial research evidence suggesting that these issues are, after all, common around the world, led us to this enhanced international publication in the English language.

We are grateful to NHS.UK for giving us the permission to reproduce parts of their guide for fussy eaters. Also, our sincere thanks go to professionals and readers who made recommendations for improvement and contributed with valuable information and ideas.

We hope you will find it helpful; all comments and suggestions are welcome.

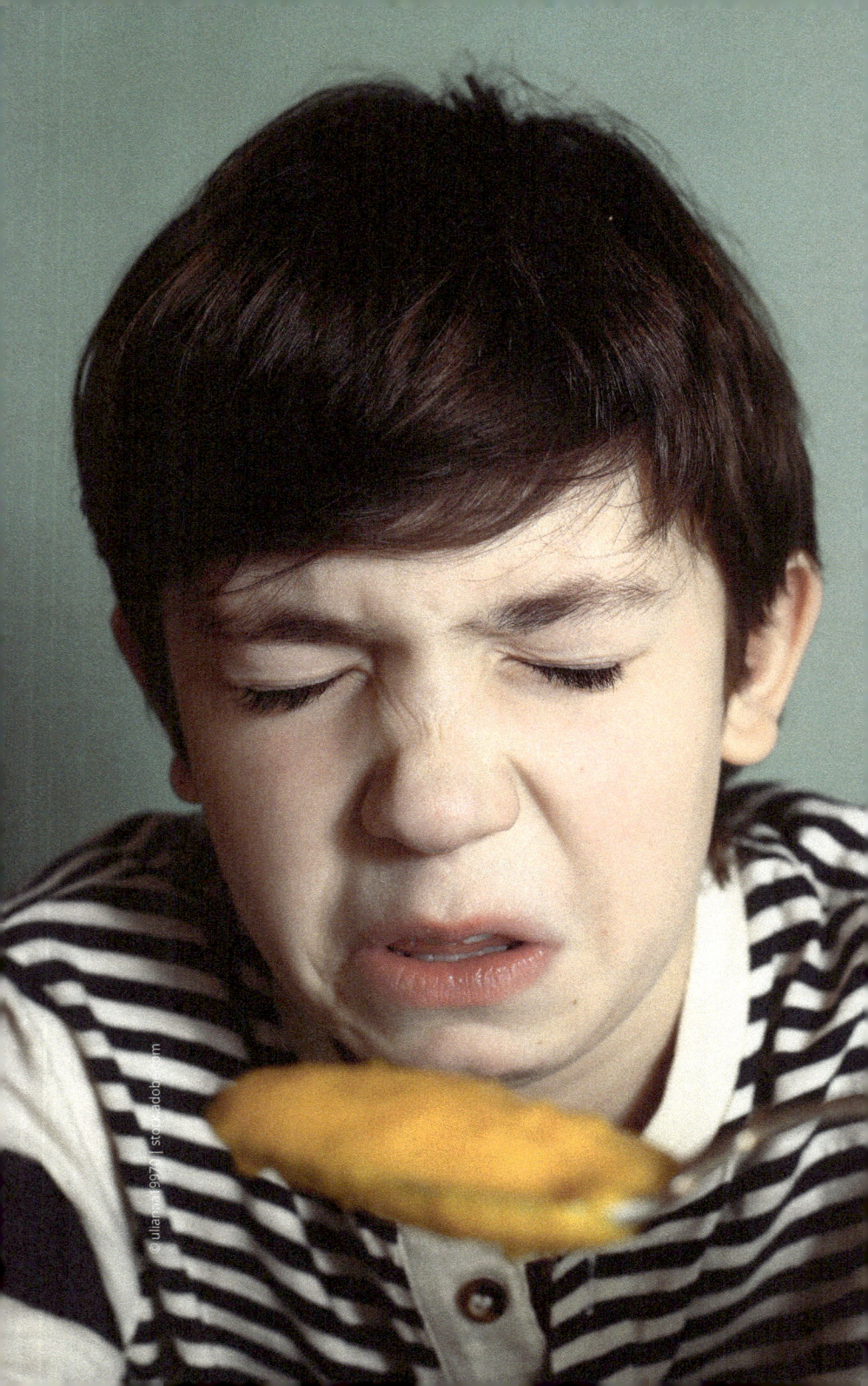

Abbreviations

- **°C:** Celsius: A scale of temperature. E.g., 180°C or 180° Celcius. 1 °Celcius= 33.8 °Fahrenheit (°F).

- **Cup:** A measure of capacity used in cooking, equal to half a US pint (0.237 litre) (North American).

- **g:** Gram (also gramme). A metric unit of mass equal to 1/1000 of a kilogram.

- **HDL:** high-density lipoprotein (good cholesterol)

- **kg:** kilogram (also kilogramme). A unit of mass, equivalent to 1000 Grams (approximately 2.205 lb).

- **lb:** Pound. A unit of weight equal to 16 oz. avoirdupois (0.4536 kg), or 12 oz. troy (0.3732 kg).

- **LDL:** low-density lipoprotein (bad cholesterol).

- **NPE:** Non-picky eater

- **tbsp:** tablespoonful (also tbs). In the UK considered to be 15 millilitres when used as a measurement in cooking.

- **tsp:** teaspoonful. In the UK considered to be 5 millilitres when used as a measurement in cooking.

See also Glossary (page 124)

Characteristics of picky eaters

Selected characteristics of children aged 1 to 5 years

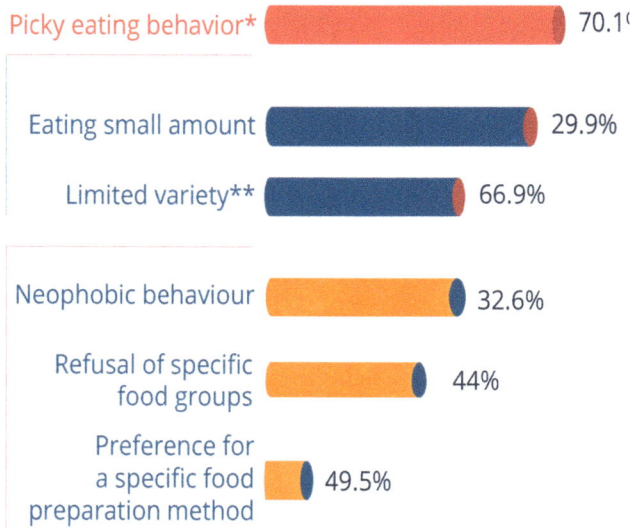

Picky eating behavior*	70.1%
Eating small amount	29.9%
Limited variety**	66.9%
Neophobic behaviour	32.6%
Refusal of specific food groups	44%
Preference for a specific food preparation method	49.5%

Sample: 184

* Children who had any one of the picky eating constructs: 'eating small amounts' and 'limited variety'.
** Children who had any one of the sub-constructs of limited variety: 'neophobic behaviour', 'refusal to eat specific food groups', and 'preference for a specific food preparation method'.

Figure 2: Kwon, K., Shim, J., Kang, M. and Paik, H.-Y. (2017). Association between Picky Eating Behaviours and Nutritional Status in Early Childhood: Performance of a Picky Eating Behaviour Questionnaire. *Nutrients*

See Glossary (page 124), references (page 138) and page 123

Introduction

If you are reading this book, there is a good chance you may feel challenged by a child's eating behaviour.

What is a fussy or a picky eater? Is there a difference with neophobia? Yes, there is.

What is the primary root of the problem? Parents' behaviour and their relationship with their children.

Do you know that if you change the colours and taste, with appropriate preparation, of the main foods that are usually rejected by picky children, the same children will eat them up?

These are only some of the topics covered in the following chapters of this guide: Fundamental rules for parents to obtain and increase skills in building consistent and straightforward behaviours in their children with delicacies and children-friendly decorated dishes.

Parents' anxiety control and their knowledge about the phenomenon and its types and what is normal or not remain a key. Because the solution requires knowledge of the problem for the parent to ask for help promptly from a doctor who is the on y person and professional that can help solve this issue.

This is the goal of this guide which covers eating difficulties from toddler age through to adolescence in five sections.

Furthermore, this book provides supplementary information from the National Health Service in the UK (NHS Choices), a detailed list of updated academic research studies, references, and a bibliography.

Abbreviations at the front end of the book, relative information, a list of recommended further reading at the end of each chapter or section, a glossary, a detailed list of references, and a bibliography aim to enhance your reading experience.

Section 1

Advice from the experts.

Causes and common mistakes members of the family make and practical advice to solve them.

© 4frame group | stock.adobe.com

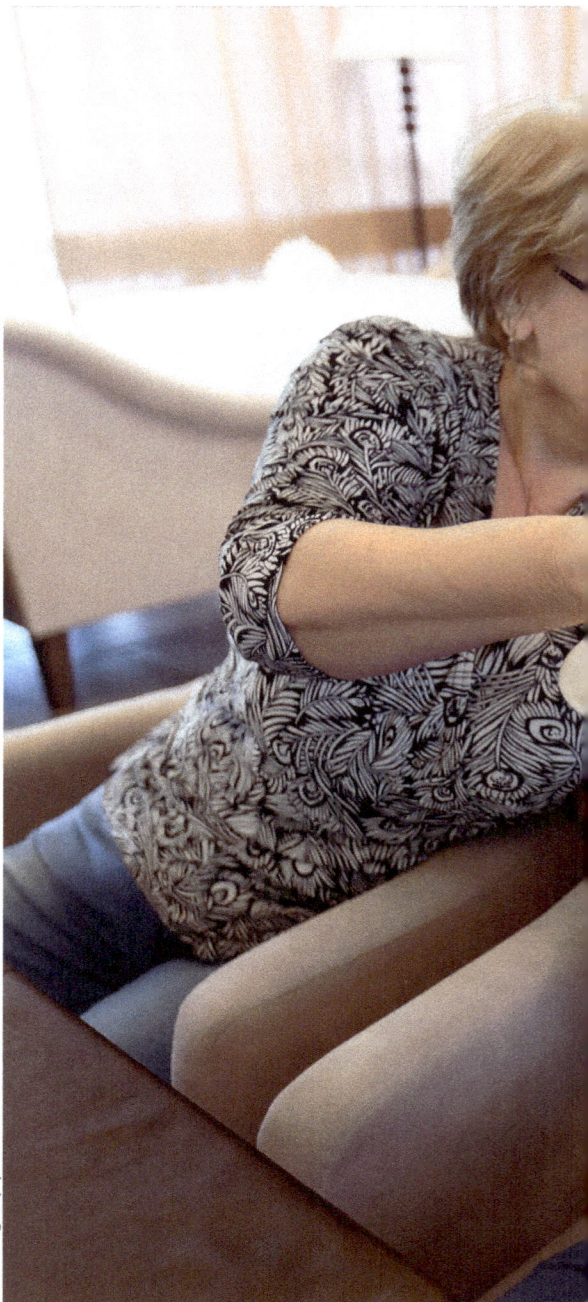

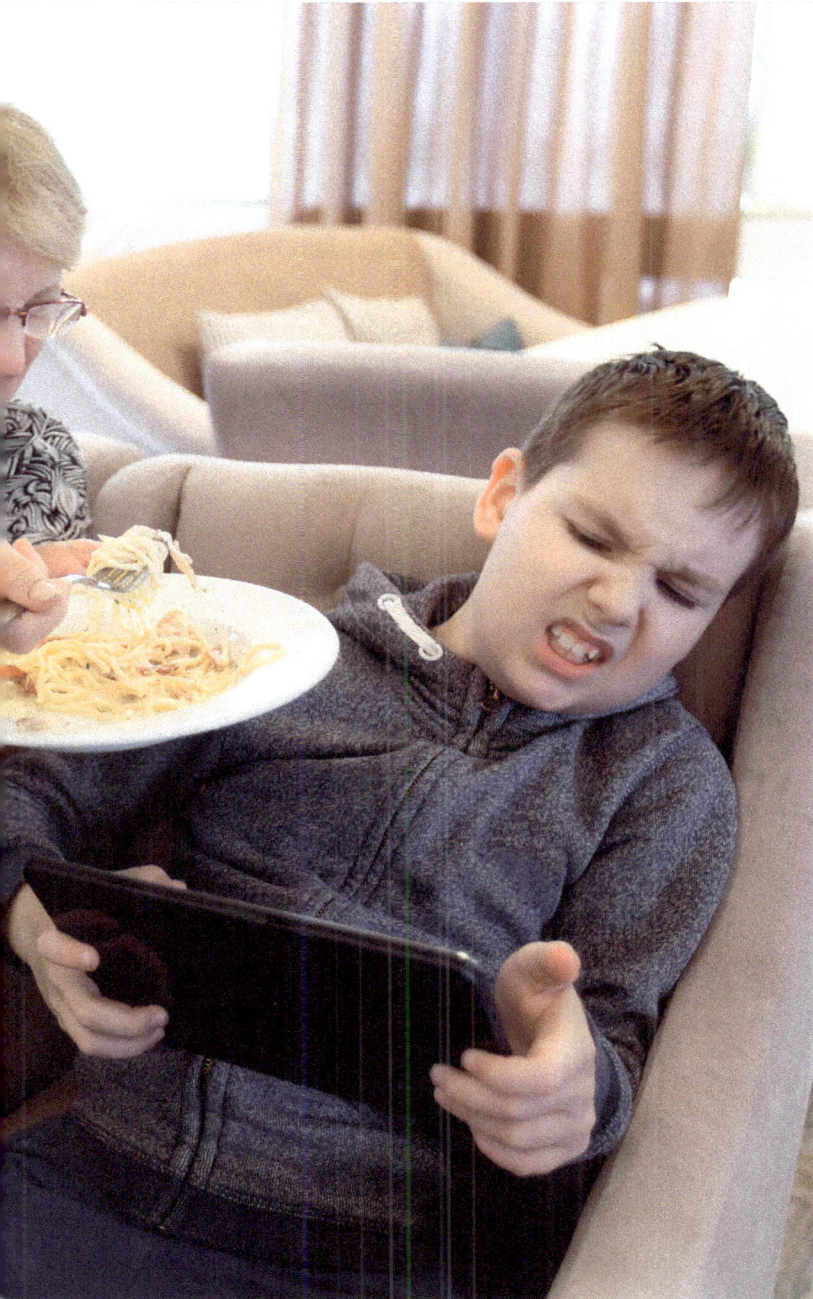

The child who refuses to eat

The power game and the danger of anorexia nervosa

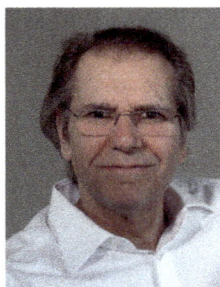

**PAVLOS
SAKKAS**
PROFESSOR OF
PSYCHIATRY AT
NATIONAL AND
KAPODISTRIAN
UNIVERSITY OF
ATHENS

Photo:
Efstratios Havaletzis

Let me start with a confession. Up to the age of 16, I was a skinny and miserable child. My parents had to run after me to make me eat. I recall that eating was a torture for me. I can't forget the times when I couldn't swallow the food that was in my mouth. I used to drink water to ease it down, but that lump of food was stuck in my throat. While I was living a nightmare, people around me kept shouting at me to get on with my eating.

It goes without saying that I had excluded many foods from my menu, while my father had tried on me all kinds of medicines that supposedly stimulated the appetite. One thing for certain was that neither my parents' efforts nor the pressure they put on me did any good. For my part, I remember dreaming of the day when a pill would be invented and save me from this torture of daily meals.

Torture described best my feelings toward eating and mainly toward the procedure of preparing meals. For my parents, though, it was agony they felt out of concern for my growth and health. Without realising it, both parties had been caught up in a disastrous power game, its epicentre being my plate. My mind filled with awe at the sight of the food heaped on my plate. It felt as if I had to climb Mount Everest, while my parents were happy with each and every mouthful that diminished the food. And when I dared to mutter "I don't want any more", they never failed to reply in chorus that the last bites were "my strength". As you can well imagine, the torture of the meal lasted a very long time. I would sit for hours in front of the plate and brood over the reasons for this parental oppression.

All children with a problematic relationship to eating tend to perceive the eating process as oppression from their parents. It is a conflict in which children have the upper hand—a conflict that allows them to take revenge for all the oppression they suffer, or what in their little minds passes for oppression, in the hands of their parents.

Taking this as a given, we may comprehend how easy it is for a child to get carried away on this dangerous road, carrying also the parents along. It is worth keeping in mind that each infant is born without any restriction as far as its expression and its behaviour are concerned. The baby does not exert any sort of control over its sphincter; it cries when in discomfort, and it cries when it is hungry. The environment that looks after it takes care of all its needs with the ultimate goal of keeping it content and quiet.

This period that Freud named "infantile omnipotence" is interrupted by the environment's gradually requiring that the baby adjusts and conforms to the

Picky eaters are "born" or "made"?

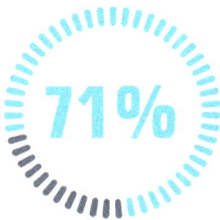

71%

2,232 respondents; 18 years and older (USA)

Fig. 3: Harris Interactive
© Statista 2018

5

conditions and the rules that have been set down. Adjustment is a long process that is carried out mainly by the parents. It is the parents who will try to help the baby and the infant adjust to the conditions that run the society in which the child is expected to live on its own sometime in the future. Later, this task is taken up by the school, where teachers and other professionals in child-rearing do their best.

Parents must override their love for their child and find the strength to educate their child.

Parents have to be fully aware of the task that society has placed on their shoulders so that they function without feelings of guilt and remorse for the restrictions — which grow gradually more and more severe — they will have to impose on their offspring. They must override their love for their child and find the strength to educate him or her, anticipating the restrictions that will be put in place by life itself. This is why a fully grown and independent individual has to eat at certain hours and at certain places; the person has to be able to control his or her sphincter muscles and carry out all biological functions within a certain framework in the appropriate manner.

A recent study (Podlesak et al., 2017) found a relationship between parenting style, parents' behaviour and picky eaters. According to the survey, "authoritarian and permissive parenting styles were positively correlated with child behaviours associated with picky eating and parent mealtime strategies that can negatively influence child feeding". In other words, some parents adopt reliable methods to overcome feeding difficulties.

Why are parents anxious about their children nutrition, and what is the appropriate approach?

Being able to provide one's body with the necessary calories from any foods is an exercise in self-sufficiency for any individual. This is one of the tasks society demands that parents complete—to teach their children to eat everything and to be able, if the need arises, to widen the range of the foods they can consume. Furthermore, insisting that their children should learn to eat all the food that is available is not a parent's foible. Therefore, parents should not be tormented by guilty feelings, provided, of course, that this education does not serve as leverage for conflicts on other fronts. Sadly, what usually happens is this: during the eating procedure, conflicts from other fronts are aired.

Sadly, this is what usually happens: during the eating procedure, there are conflicts with other fronts that exist.

For instance, a child may well refuse to eat a certain food or skip an entire meal in protest against the parent who did not allow the child to watch television. While the example of the television is quite obvious to the parent, in some other cases, the parent is totally unaware of the fact that the child perceives the parent's refusal as rejection. In this case, the child, for example, might ask for physical contact, like a hug or a caress, which the parent might refuse at this specific time. This refusal might be negligible for the parent; for the child, however, it could signal a conflict, which of course will be carried on to a field where the child can exert advantageous power. Unfortunately, such fields for the child are intense crying, going to bed late, sphincter control, and of course, eating. As the child grows older, the list grows, too: misconduct, mischief, and refusal to study for school.

If we do not promptly treat the problem, i.e., the restoration of the relationship between parents and children, the catastrophic behaviour for the child will continue, and take different forms throughout his life. Moreover, eating difficulties can remain. Kown et al. (2017) say that "If food neophobia [refusal of tasting and introducing new foods] "it is not appropriately countered at the period of introduction of complementary food, some food groups may remain refused throughout [his/her] life."

I often say that children are perverts because, being determined to hurt their parent, they are willing to disregard their discomfort, even their pain.

I often say that children are perverts because, being determined to hurt their parent, they are willing to disregard their own discomfort, even their own pain. They may be hungry, but they are patient in order for them to punish the parent by upsetting him or her. Believe me, children perceive better than any adult the parent's feelings. Recognising the feelings of those around us is a skill we have as babies, long before we learn how to decode the words used for communication by the people close to us. Just like a dog can tell from the intensity and the tone of our voice and our body language what we want it to understand, babies and infants feel what hurts their parents and caretakers. It is easy for children to find our weak spots, and once they do, they know where to strike if they have to.

It goes without saying that in the long procedure of teaching our children, conflicts will inevitably arise, so it is crucial that we don't let our weaknesses show early. Keeping a tight rein on our agonies is important when, just once, our child refuses a certain kind of food or even refuses to eat. The same goes for the other fronts where the child has the upper hand. Stripped of sentimentalities and guilt feelings, the parent has to put up with the child's efforts to bring about conflict, using loud crying and shouting, suspension of sphincters control, ostentatious mischief or, finally, difficulties in eating. Self-restraint and suspension of emotion from the part of the parents and the caretakers are the keys for avoiding these fields of advantages for the children conflict.

Self-restraint and suspension of emotion from the part of the parents and the caretakers are the keys to avoiding these fields of advantage for conflict with children.

It is essential to avoid implicating oneself in these fields of conflict that end up in psychic and physical wear and tear for both parties. Naturally it is the child that pays the heavier, most tangible price, though the price the parents have to pay is also hard to ponder. Once the family takes this road, it is difficult to call a halt. Sometimes other aspects of the relationships between the members of the family may emerge. You may often find that once on this particular road, a game of guilt between the parents might ensue, which may end up in even more serious conflicts between the two. A fussy child may well tear a family apart. Let us always keep in mind that family is an institution that takes a lot of effort to keep together. A fussy child may either reinforce the ties of coherence, or, quite the opposite, intensify the centrifugal forces.

The only way to stop going downhill is the disentanglement of the parents from this conflict. I strongly recommend that the parents remain firm and not allow their children's foibles upset them. It's best to admit their defeat and draw back from the conflict. As a matter of fact, this requires absolute concurrence between the parents. It's no good when one parent does not care while the other does their best to persuade the child to eat or study. Seeing eye to eye on a guilt-free basis is a prerequisite for their reaction in this graceless conflict with the child. They have to side-step the game of putting the blame for the family to defeat each other. Moreover, nobody knows who made the first mistake and at what point the control over the relationship with the child was lost.

A game of guilt between the parents might ensue, which may end up in even more serious conflicts between the two.

Initially, the child will perceive this withdrawal from the conflict by the parents as temporary strategic tactics, aiming to entrap it in the result they desire. It is to be expected that the child will almost certainly persist in the tactics of his or her choice.

Power game

The parents will have to be firm in their decision to withdraw until the child is convinced that the parents mean what they say. This is the crucial point of the game – the climax of the power game that started some years ago and developed into a psychopathological condition for the child and into a family drama in general.

At this critical point, the parents just have to keep their cool to show to the child that they are no longer going to interfere in their child's deviating – in their opinion – behaviour. Only then shall the child change his or her ways, when it is certain that blackmail will not manipulate the parents anymore. It will be very hard for the parents to sit back and watch their child self-destruct; to refrain from reacting like they used to.

This is the only, albeit dangerous, way to exit the vicious circle of this pointless conflict. Yes, I do admit that this is dangerous for the child, particularly if he or she perseveres or if the parents are not firm and show signs of going back to previous behaviour. These signs are perceived by the child as weakness and as going back on their word which results in an eternal repetition of a pathological and destructive tug of war.

It will be tough for the parents to sit back and watch their child self-destruct and to refrain from reacting, like they used to do in the past.

I don't mean to scare parents, but as far as the conflict over eating is concerned, they should be aware of, in extreme cases, the danger of anorexia nervosa. As described in my book, *Revealing psychiatry... from an insider* (Sakkas, 2015) it may lead to a not so negligible number of deaths in children. Undoubtedly, it is much better to pre-empt conflict over the plate than trying to correct post hoc psychopathology.

Let it be noted at this point that conflict over the plate is not always enacted by the pair parents and child; it might often concern the conflict between the parents themselves or even the caretakers, meaning that sometimes one parent offers the child a food that the other one prohibits. In this way the breach in the relationship between the parents or between one parent and one care-taker (grandma, granddad, uncle, aunt, or other family member) is intensified by the child's behaviour. And let us not forget what I noted previously, that children are perverted, meaning that they enjoy the disruption they cause to their environment.

As far as a conflict about eating is concerned, in extreme cases, the lurking danger of anorexia nervosa exists. This situation may lead to a not-so-negligible number of children's death.

A milder approach to an established pathological relationship between a child and food is exactly the subject of this book. In other words, how will the child achieve a normal interaction with foods, without having to take the parents out of the picture? Furthermore, in what way is the relationship between parent and child over a heaped plate going to be restored? To sum it up, this book aims to serve as a roadmap to eating normalcy, minus the crying and the emotional extremities.

Coming back full circle, I will close with a personal experience, just like I started. My interaction with eating was restored, as if by magic, when at the age of 16 I was sent abroad on a camping holiday. There, away from my parents, I was forced to compete with other children my age. I had to compare myself to them, away from the protection of the family, where my sentimental blackmails to my parents counted for absolutely nothing.

I do hope that this chapter will help not only restore children's relationship with eating, but what is more, prevent it from being disrupted.

Interesting to read

Dealing with child behaviour problems

By NHS.UK Choices (Appendix 1, page 125)

Make your child love food

Falsities and truths about "good" and "bad" foods

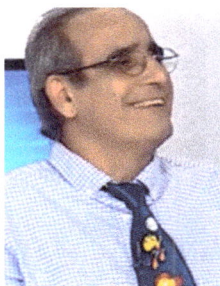

GEORGE MOUSTAKAS

PAEDIATRICIAN

When I was asked to contribute to the writing of this book with my experiences as a paediatrician, the first thing that came to mind was the comparison between food and the medicines we give to children.

Medicines are a necessary evil that we have to take in order to recover from an illness, whereas food is indispensable to our growth and our healthy development. Food, just like medicine, has to be characterized by some adjectives (tasty, attractive) so that our children will take it without much fuss.

The main reason for rejecting foods are distaste and dislike of colour, according to studies by Addessi et al. (2005) and Koivisto et al. (1996). Also, studies showed "that an appropriate food preparation method that positively influences food intake would be helpful for the prevention of poor growth" (Kwon et al. 2017).

Well, how can we make food attractive and tasty?

Taste: We know that man uses his senses in order for him to enjoy food, so I thought it would be worth it to refer to these senses a little more extensively; these senses are touch (somatosensation), sight (vision), smell (olfaction), taste (gustation), and the sixth sense, known as intuition.

Smell: Children, from quite a young age, can tell the difference between tastes and react accordingly showing their pleasure or displeasure; this is why the food we serve them should be neither too bitter nor too salty, neither too sweet and nor too sour. In other words, the food should have a well-balanced taste.

Touch: The smell should be pleasing because lots of children first smell the food and then eat it. Therefore, a bad smell is an inhibiting and repelling factor that does not allow them to bring food closer and eat.

Sight: Children love eating with their hands, the sense of touch is very important to them. Therefore we should avoid food that is hard or gluey, as well as those with fuzz or thorns.

Intuition: The way we present food is also important. Therefore, we place small portions on the plate, using various ingredients, in different colours and shapes like, for example, smiley faces, so that food becomes appealing and pleasing.

When we set a plate on the table, a child's mind automatically processes all that is perceived through its senses (like the tone of our voice, the expression on our face, our body posture), and using thus its intuition, the child accepts or rejects the food.

Interesting to read

Fussy eaters: Tips for parents

By NHS Choices (Appendix 2, *page 128*)

No panic!

Almost every day, we meet anxious parents with picky eater kids. It is a widespread phenomenon in children. Paediatric providers should support parents in expanding the number of healthy foods children eat to improve dietary quality but reassure parents that picky eating is not associated with children's weight status or micronutrient deficiencies (Brown et al. 2018). However, the medium and long-term impacts have not been thoroughly investigated; and, therefore, there are disagreements (Kwon et al., 2017; Mascola et al. 2017).

However, the majority of studies have not concluded to significant effects on growth were observed.

Necessary ingredients for children's health that also make foods tastier.

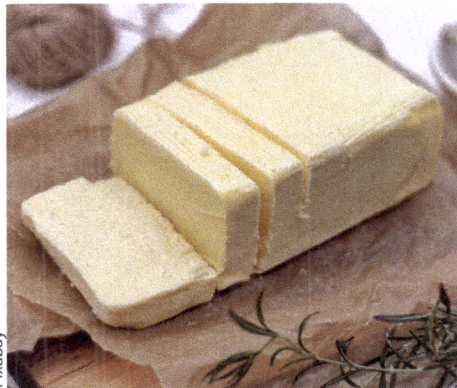

Pixabay

Butter

What to feed young children

By NHS.
UK Choices
(Appendix 3,
page 130)

Raw butter contains vitamins A and E, selenium, and iodine, which help the thyroid gland, the suprarenal glands, and the heart in their functions. It is rich in good cholesterol, which is called high-density lipoprotein (HDL). HDL is necessary for the development of the nervous system and brain. It also contains vitamin K2, which prevents dental caries, and contributes to the good health of teeth and bones.

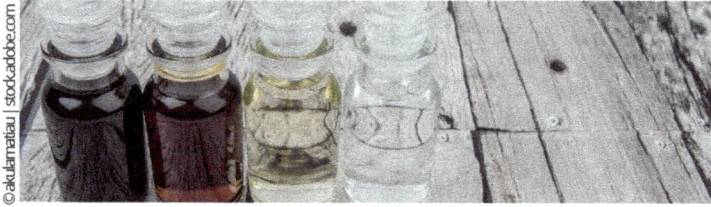

Vinegar

Vinegar, apart from adding taste to food, is quite an effective medicine. We have balsamic, red, and white vinegar.

It is made of grapes, apples, fruits, tomatoes, walnuts, pulses, and rice. The ones that taste best are those made of grapes and apple (apple vinegar). Hippocrates had referred to its therapeutic properties, especially for pain in the joints, digestive problems, and blood disorders.

Most parents use it to make fever go down by placing a rug soaked in a water and vinegar solution on the child's forehead. However, vinegar can do much more than that: it helps decongest the respiratory system and relieve a sore throat, relieves headaches, soothes pain from burns and prevents the formation of blisters, soothes the pain and itch from insect bites (mosquitoes, bees), stops yeast infection of the toes, drives away lice (by combing hair with water and vinegar), and removes stains from cherries, beetroot, and berries from the hands.

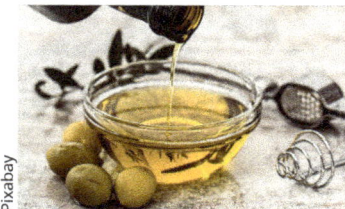

Olive oil

The ancient Greeks used to call virgin olive oil "liquid gold." It is rich in fatty acids, decreases LDL (bad cholesterol) thus protecting the heart, and fights constipation, whereas as an anti-oxidant, it flushes the toxins through the liver and gall bladder, and as an anti-inflammatory, it fights pain in the joints and furthermore strengthens the hair and protects from dry skin.

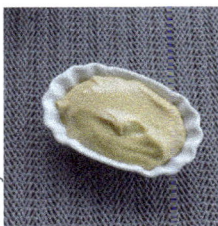
Pixabay

Mustard

It contains selenium, magnesium, B complex vitamins, as well as vitamins A, C, and K. It lowers cholesterol and soothes asthma crises and common cold; it also relieves muscular pain.

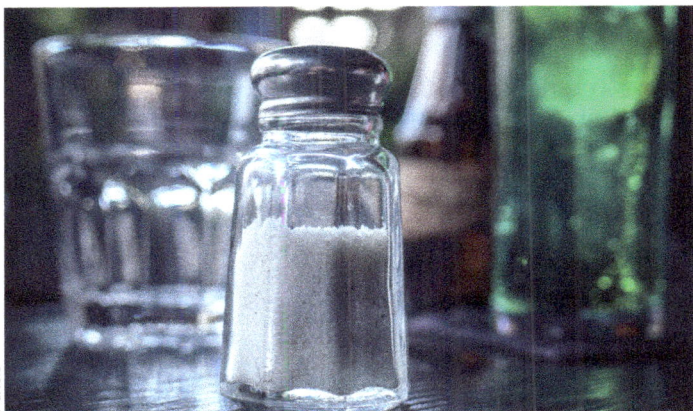
Pexels

Salt

Natural sea salt prevents cramps and night drooling in children. It is also a natural powerful antihistaminic. It can cure catarrh (a runny nose) and congestion; it strengthens the bones, helps with better sleep, helps the intestine absorb trace elements, and helps the cleansing of the lungs of mucus (particularly useful for children with mucoviscidosis and asthma). Furthermore it helps blood sugar levels balance, stabilizes heart rate, regulates blood pressure, and provides energy to our cells.

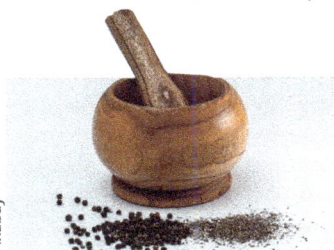
Pixabay

Pepper

Pepper adds taste to food and helps with digestion.

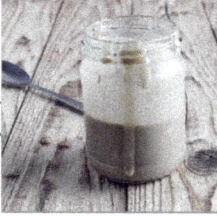

© Alex Bayev | Adobe Stock

Tahini

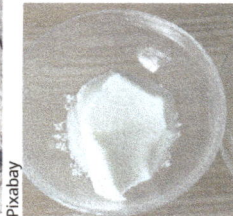

Pixabay

Yoghurt

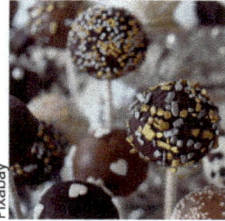

Pixabay

Chocolate

Tahini contains calcium, phosphorus, potassium, magnesium, copper, iron, a natural protein of high biological value, omega 6, vitamin E, and carbohydrates. It helps the normal function of the digestive system, reduces cholesterol and helps the bones develop properly.

It is rich in protein of a high biological value, also high in calcium, phosphorus, zinc, iodine, vitamins A and B. It helps re-establish intestinal flora balance (it is prescribed to individuals who are on antibiotics, where the intestinal flora is destroyed).

Chocolate is quite beneficial, particularly the dark variety. It lowers cholesterol, regulates blood pressure, boosts brain functions, smooths the epidermis, relieves intense coughing, regulates blood sugar, and enhances eyesight.

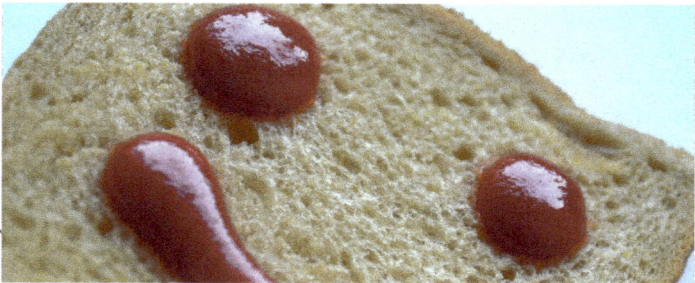

Pixabay

Ketchup

This foodstuff is made of tomato. It is rich in vitamin A, which is essential for healthy eyes, skin, teeth and bones. It also contains lycopene, which keeps cholesterol at the desired levels in our blood and at the same time reduces bad cholesterol.

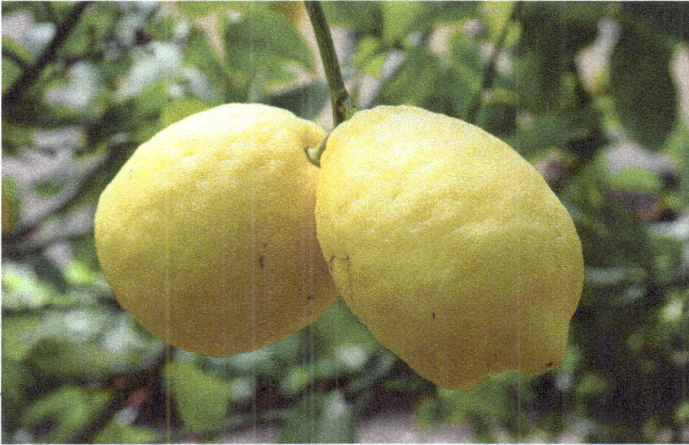

Pixabay

Lemon

Adds taste to tasteless, colourless and uninteresting food stuff. It's juice contains a high amount of vitamins C, B1, B2, B3 and B6, protein, carbohydrates, potassium, calcium, magnesium and minerals. It protects organisms from certain illnesses and inflammation (virus, flu, cold). It is an anti-oxidant and it also reduces blood pressure (through potassium). It helps reduce high fever and it also has antimicrobial and antibacterial properties, particularly in relation to the throat and tonsils. Furthermore, it can be used locally on insect and jellyfish bites, it relieves toothache, and it acts as a haemostatic agent (a piece of cotton wool dipped in lemon juice and placed in the nose stops nosebleeds). It acts as an antidote for food poisoning from seafood and shellfish. It helps in the absorption of iron and calcium and fights constipation by cleansing the intestine and reinforcing peristalsis. Finally, it cures scurvy.

However, let us not forget that everything has to be used in moderation. Like our ancestors used to say: "Moderation is the best thing".
Always follow your doctor's advice in case of a pathological issue that may require a specific diet.

Parents should start gradually introducing their children to different tastes from the age of 6 to 12 months—for example, potatoes, carrots, zucchini, broccoli, spinach, tomatoes, rand onions from the vegetable group and apples, pears, bananas, kiwifruits, and apricots from the fruit group. It is crucial to find the right trick to make children eat as it has been noted that a trick that works with one child may not work with another, even for children in the same family. It doesn't matter which trick the parents will use to achieve their goal because, in the end, it is the result that matters.

1 We cook together

We ask our children to participate in the preparation of the food. We should remember to make the food tastier by adding any of the above-mentioned ingredients (salt, lemon, vinegar, yogurt, tahini, mayonnaise, mustard, ketchup, chocolate, and pepper). While cooking, we ask the children to try the food for flavour and ask what has to be added or reduced in their opinion.

As the children grow up, we should include them in the entire process of the meal, right from the start, taking them with us to the market or the green grocer's and picking together the food stuff (vegetables, fruit, and whatever else is necessary). Now is the time to start adding flavour to our food with salt, pepper, lemon, vinegar, etc.

2 The joy of creation

Older children would like the task of drafting the menu of the week. We may assist them by choosing among the tasty recipes that our friend Rena tis Ftelias, after so many years in the cu inary field, has offered (see inside the book).

Reward day

3

We motivate our children to pick their favourite meal once a week, even if it is not entirely healthy.

Serving the food

4

When the cooking is done, we invite the children to take part in setting the table by choosing glasses, cutlery, paper napkins, and medium-sized plates. We try to eat all together at least twice a week, if it is possible, not in front of the television, and if it is already on, we have better turn it off before the meal starts.

The portions have to be small (keeping in mind that they are still children with a small stomach), and the dishes should be colourful, containing, for example, carrots, fresh peas, and red peppers (Nutrition Australia).

Tasting and learning about food

5

We let our child try the food from our plate because the child might believe that our food is tastier, and vice versa, we try theirs to confirm that we like it.

Ask your children to taste the foods, and accept the fact that they may not like them. If this is the case, try a different way of cooking, or add some of their favourites, i.e., carrots or meat can be put in the blender and made into a sauce for spaghetti.

6

Let the children eat on their own

We let the children eat on their own if they want to, even with their hands – why not – even if that means they will get dirty. Our goal is to make eating a happy occurrence – to make it fun!

7

No in-between snacks

We try to avoid snacks (chips, chocolate, etc.) between the meals of the day. It is better to let hunger take its toll: when the child gets sufficiently hungry, food will seem more appealing, and he or she will be more enthusiastic about eating (Nutrition Australia).

8

Imitation

Let's keep in mind that children between the age of 2 and 3 discover refusal (NO! NO! NO!) for certain foods. For example, they refuse to take salad, fruit, or milk. Do not let the fact upset you. Do not think that your children will never eat these foods. As they grow older, they will have to taste them and eat them. When they find themselves at the kindergarten, at a friend's party, at camp or an excursion, they will try these foods as long as you are the living example and eat these foods in front of the children.

9

Fruit salad

We can trick our children into eating fruits using fruit salad which we will prepare together. We let them choose two or three fruits of their liking; then we add another one, then we wash them, peel them, cut them, add a squirt of lemon, a spoonful of sugar, put it in the fridge, then serve it in the child's favourite bowl. We can also chop some fruit into the yoghurt, so in the afternoon, a refreshing, wholesome snack will be waiting for the child.

10

It is not a disease

Finally, we should know that fussy children are healthy children, not sick. It just takes patience. We have to allocate a lot of our time to play along with them; we ourselves have to become children again, in order to establish an easy communication with them. Through play our children get happy, tired and hungry; therefore, they eat with more enthusiasm.

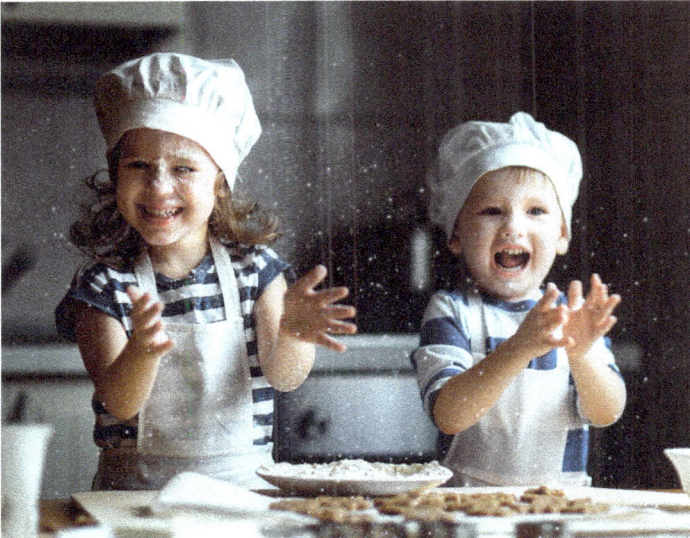

Section 2

*Delicacies
by Chef Eirini
Togia.*

---

*The goal:
make
children love
eating.*

*Pay attention
to possible
limitations
(i.e., allergies,
high
cholesterol,
diabetes). Ask
your doctor
to replace
or delete
harmful
ingredient(s).*

© vkuslandia | stock.adobe.com

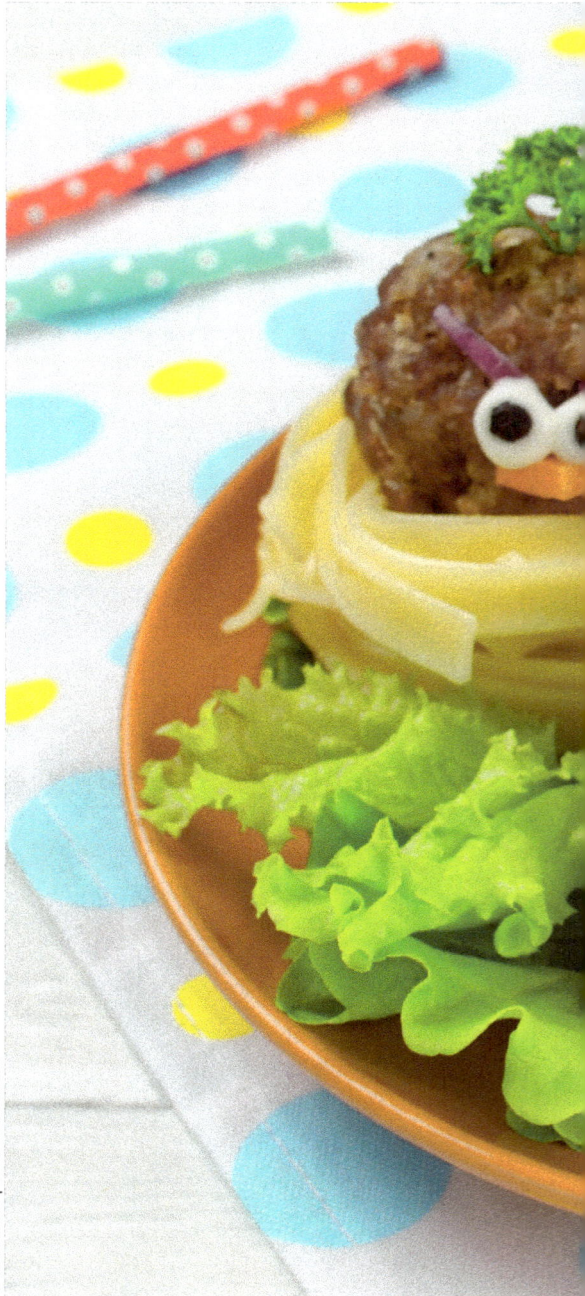

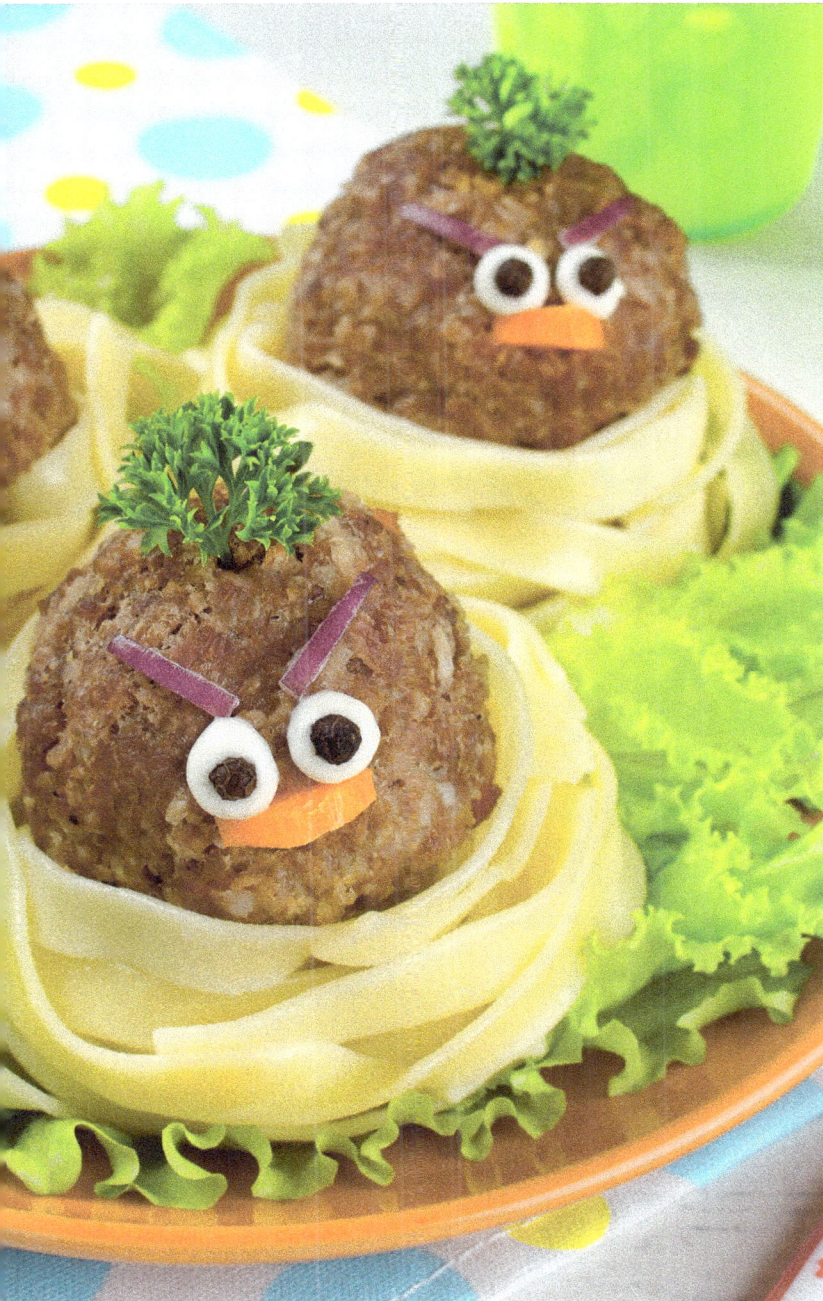

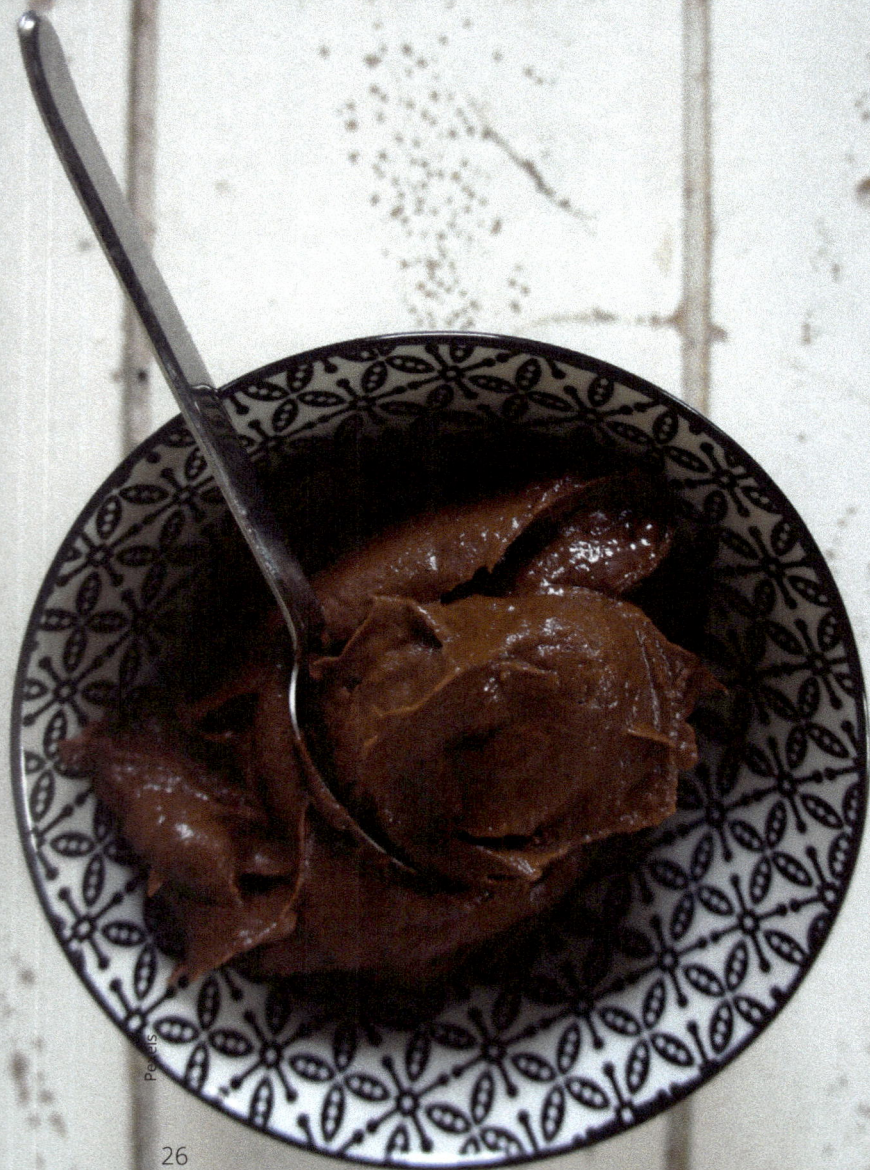

Snack

Pealis

You can keep it in the fridge for one week

Fruity choco spread

I peel the bananas and slice them, then I cut the avocados in two, take out the stone, and with a spoon, I dig out the flesh.

I put all the ingredients in the multi until I obtain a smooth, homogenous mixture. I put this in a food container, cover it with the lid, and leave it in the fridge for 2 hours.

I can use this choco spread on biscuits, cookies, bread, and crackers.

It is a different, wholesome choco spread.

Tip

If necessary, I may add 2-3 tbsp of milk while still in the multi.

INGREDIENTS

- 2 ripe bananas
- 2 ripe avocados
- 3 tbsp chicken
- 4 tbsp honey

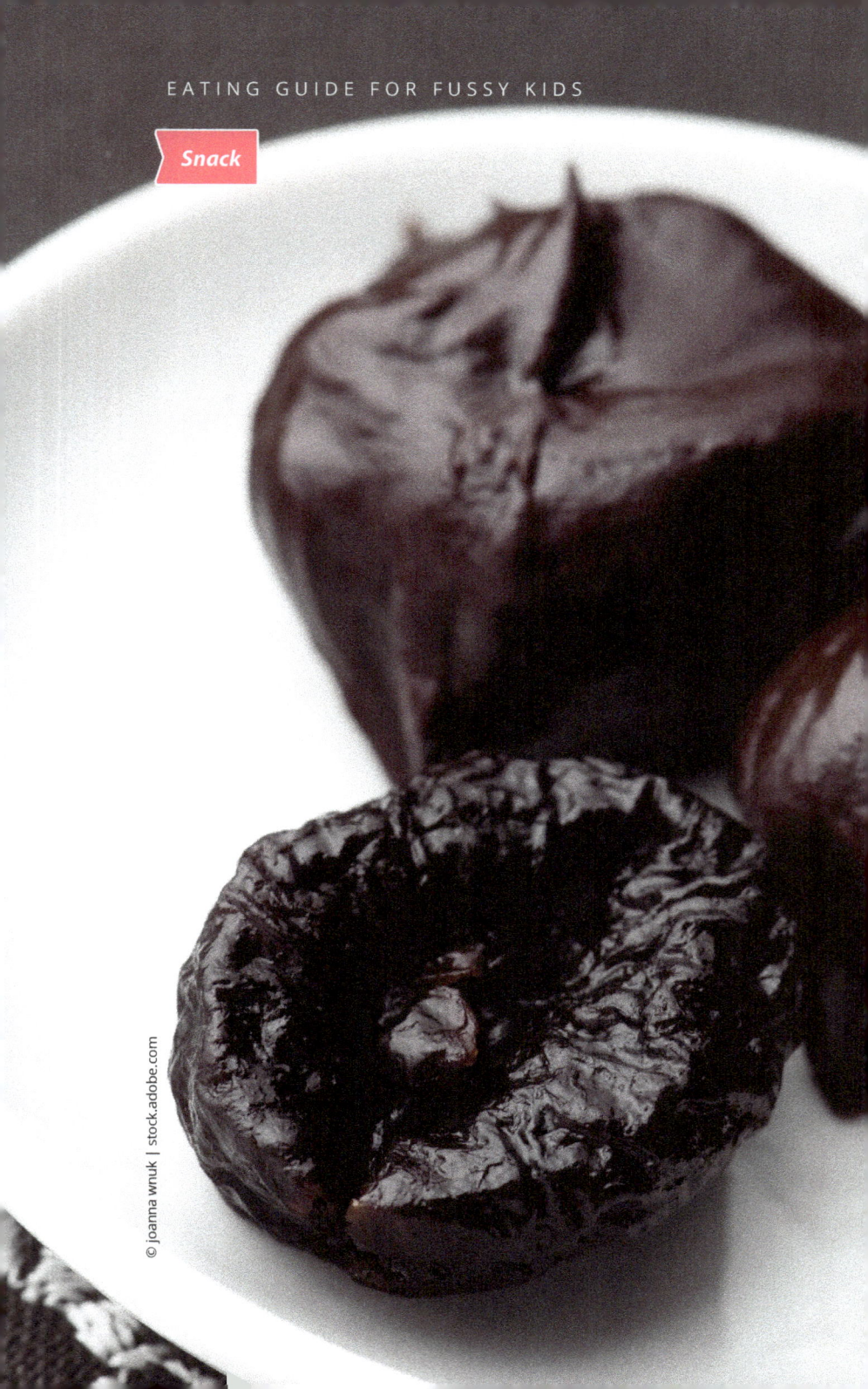

Enjoy!

Chocolate-dipped plums

I use a bain-marie[1] to melt the chocolate bars. I chop the nuts separately in the multi (5 almonds, 5 hazelnuts, 5 walnuts).

I open the plums in 2 halves and place a teaspoonful of the chopped nuts in the centre of each and then close them.

I dip each plum separately in the chocolate, then place them on baking paper and leave them to dry. When the chocolate is stable, they are ready!

Tip

I chop the nuts in the multi to make sure that it will be easier for the kids to eat them.

INGREDIENTS

- 15 plums
- 5 almonds
- 5 hazelnuts
- 5 walnuts
- 2 bars of cooking chocolate (200 g each)

---

1 *Place the chocolate in a saucepan, and place the pan in a bigger saucepan containing water up to the 1/3 of the smaller saucepan. Bring the water to a boil, thus heating the chocolate until it melts completely.*

Meal

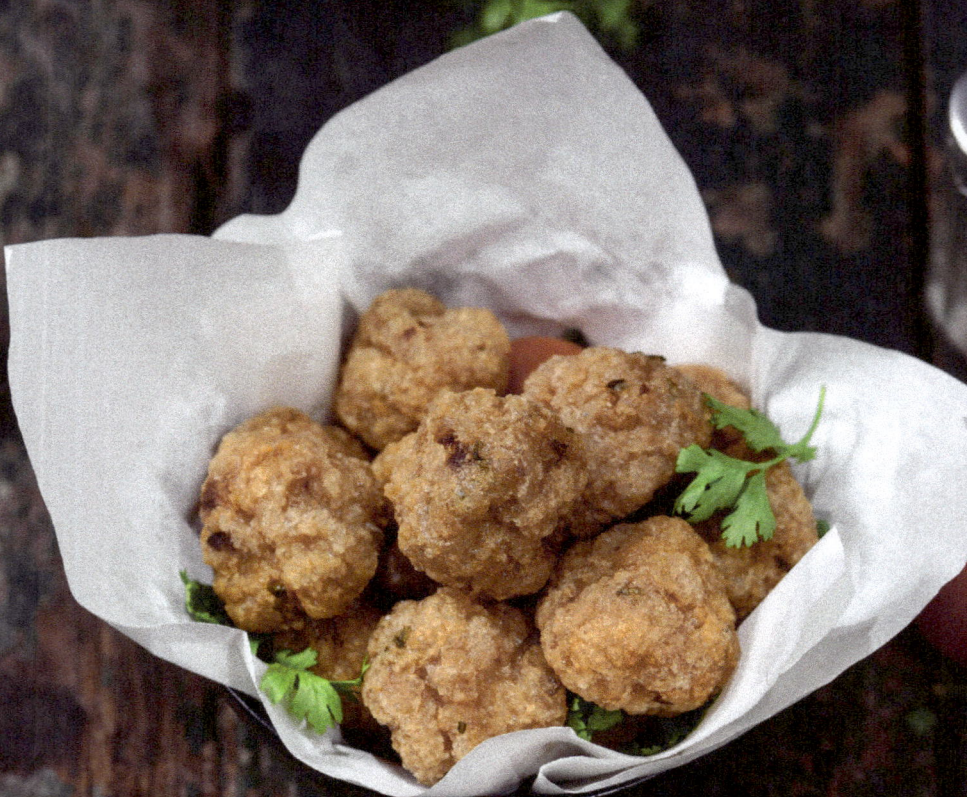

Ideal for kids who don't eat fish

Fish balls

I fill a saucepan with water up to its middle and turn up the heat. When the water boils, I add the fish slices, the sliced potatoes, and the carrots, and let them simmer. When they are done, I remove the ingredients from the water and let them cool.

I then remove all the bones very carefully from the fish. With a fork, I mash the potatoes and the carrots. In a bowl, I add the fish (cut in morsels), the mashed potatoes and carrots, the tomato, and the onion. I then add the oil and the parsley and season the mixture. I put it in the fridge for a while.

Then I bring out the mixture and pat it into small balls. On a platter, I spread out the flour and roll the balls in the flour (like meatballs). I add frying oil to the pan, and when it is sufficiently hot, I cook them, a few at a time.

Serve hot!

INGREDIENTS

- 1 kg fish slices
- 1 onion, grated
- 1 tomato
- 2 potatoes, sliced
- 1 carrot, sliced
- Parsley, finely chopped
- Salt, pepper
- 2 tbsp olive oil
- Flour
- Frying oil

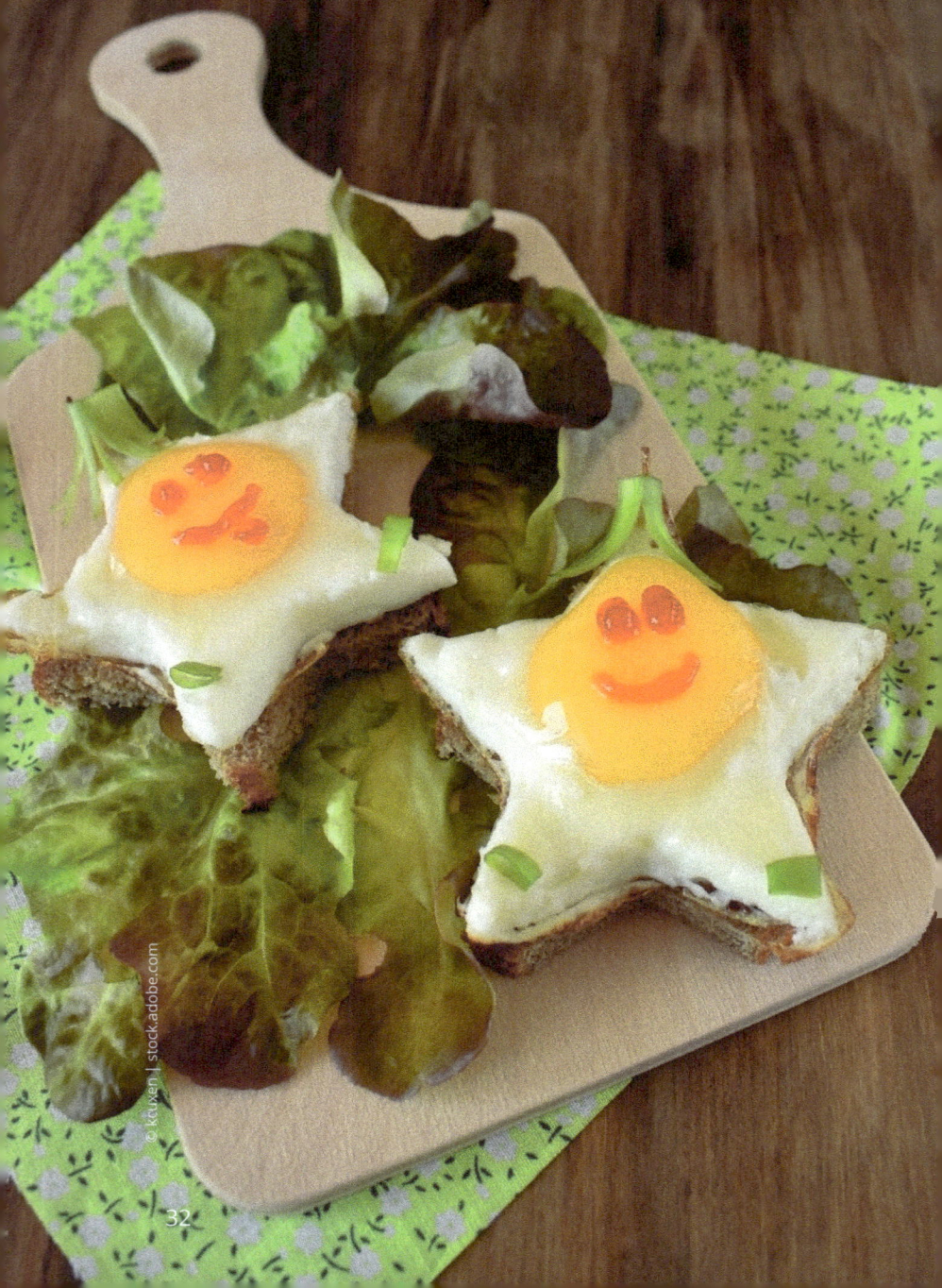

With fried egg and imagination, for more variations

Toasted smiley face

With the help of cookie cutters, I cut the bread slices into several shapes.

When the oil in the pan is hot enough, I add the bread slices one at a time.

In the same pan, I use a mould of the same shape to fry the egg so the egg is the same shape as the bread. I repeat the procedure with the remaining bread slices and eggs.

When the bread and the eggs are ready, I place them on a platter. The bread goes on the bottom, and the egg goes on top. I use the pepper and the cucumber to draw two eyes; then the carrot becomes the mouth. The result is a smiley face that encourages children to eat their eggs.

This is one way of doing it. Use your imagination and other ingredients to create more figures.

INGREDIENTS

- 6 slices of bread for toast
- 6 eggs
- 1 small cucumber cut into sticks
- 1 pepper
- 1 carrot cut into sticks
- Oil
- Salt and pepper

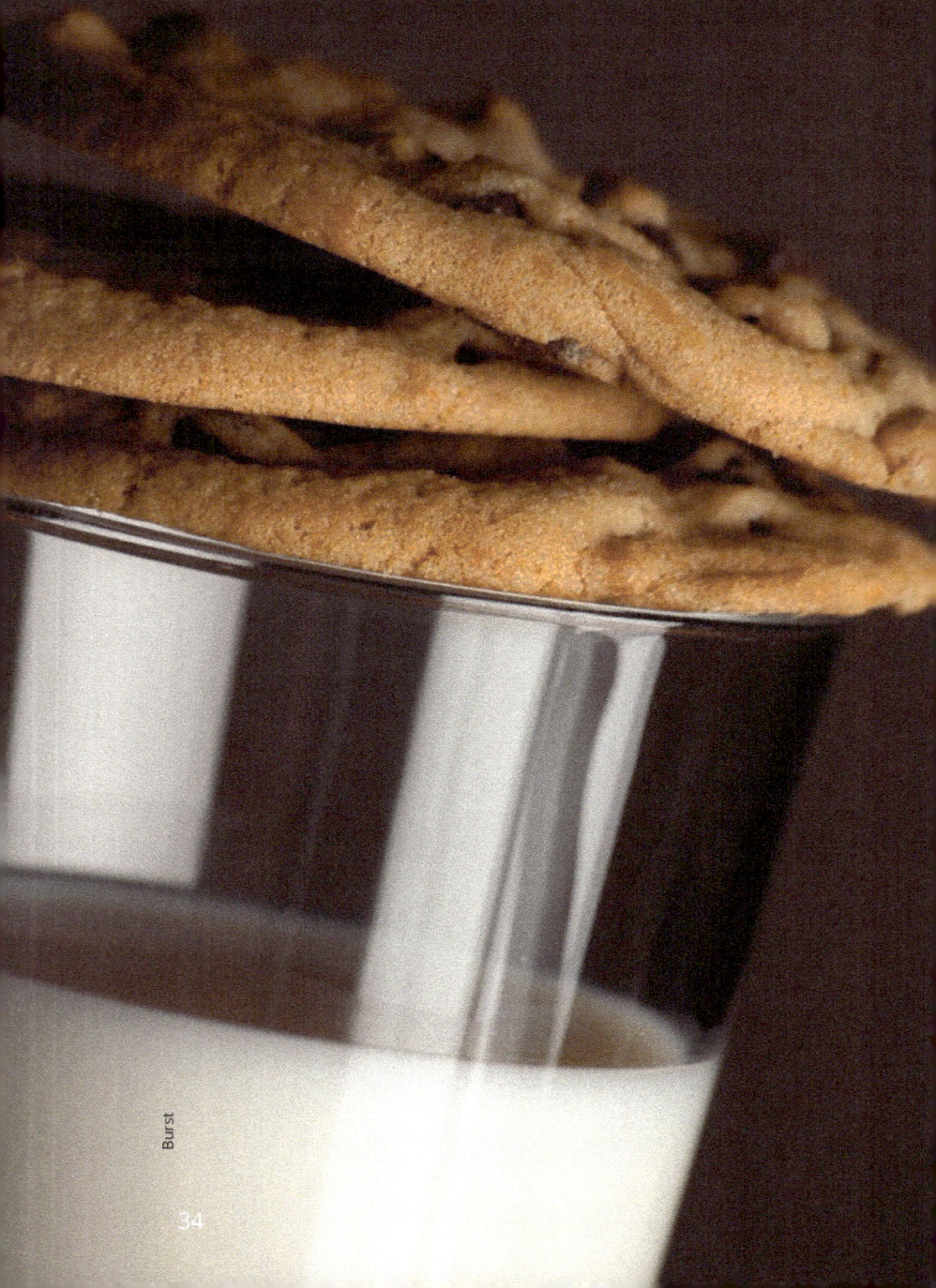

Snack

Burst

Perfect for grown-up kids too!

Chocolate cookies

First, I warm the butter until it melts. Then I mix all the ingredients in a bowl. I combine them into a soft dough.

I divide it into 2 – 3 cylinders, wrap them in cling film, and leave them in the fridge for a couple of hours.

I preheat the oven to 160° C, line an oven dish with baking paper, cut the cylinders into slices (just like bread), and place them in the oven dish. I bake them for 40-45 minutes.

It's perfect for breakfast, also ideal as an afternoon snack at the park, and for... grown up kids at the office

INGREDIENTS

- 500 g soft flour
- 1 tsp baking powder
- 250 g butter
- 200 g brown sugar
- 3 eggs
- 300 g diced chocolate
- Orange zest

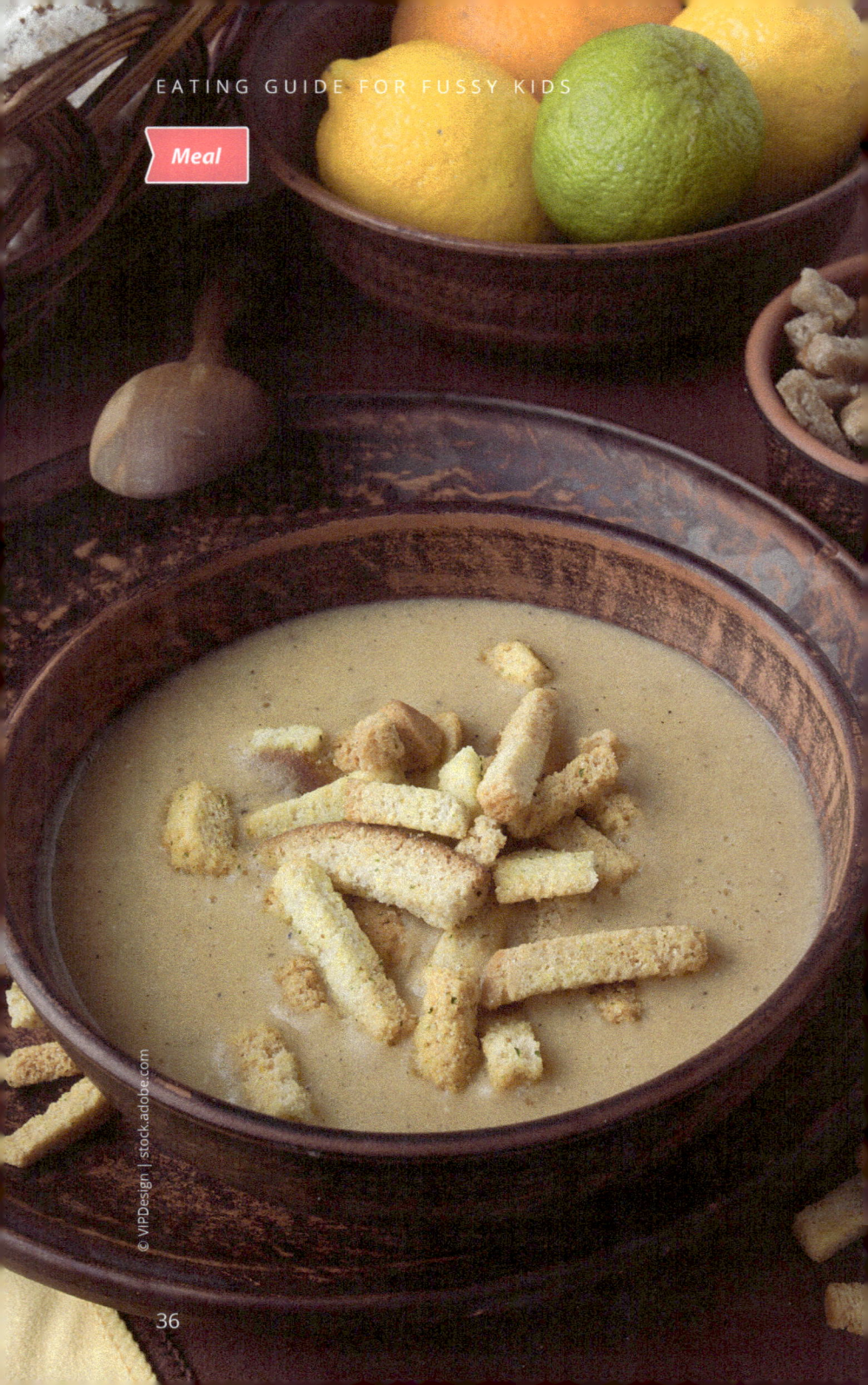

For kids who avoid pulses

Lentil mousse

I put the oil and butter in a saucepan and turn up the heat. I brown the onion, the leeks, and the carrots for 4-5 minutes. Then I add the lentils, the bay leaves, 3 glasses of water, and salt and pepper and bring it all to a simmer until the fluid thickens.

While still in the saucepan beat the ingredients with a hand blender to a nice smooth cream.

It is delicious, and the lentils are not detectable. A perfect way to make kids eat lentils!

INGREDIENTS

- 200 g lentils
- 200 g diced carrots
- 100 g diced leeks
- 1 onion, diced
- 2-3 bay leaves
- 3 tbsp butter
- 3 tbsp oil
- Salt, pepper

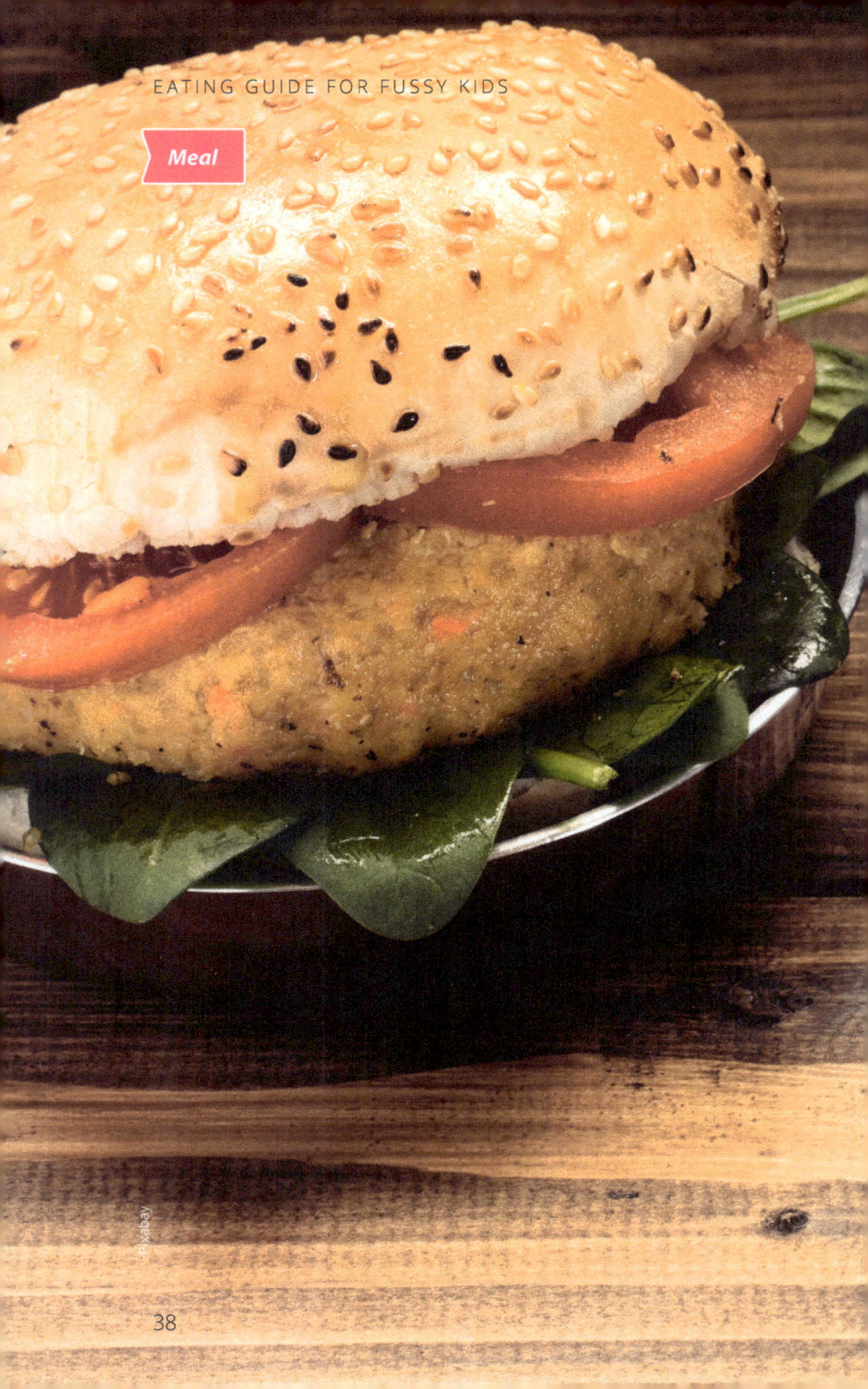

Meal

For children who avoid vegetables

Veggie burgers

Preheat the oven to 180° C.

Strain the boiled vegetables thoroughly and put them in a bowl.

Then, add the parsley, mint, tomato, and breadcrumbs and mix them all very well. Cover with cling film and put the mixture in the fridge for one hour. Grease the oven dish with oil. Pat the mixture into small burgers or balls and place them in the dish. Roast them for 15 minutes, then turn them over and roast for another 10 minutes.

As an option, add yellow cheese slices on top of each burger at the final roasting phase, and it will melt.

The kids will love their veggies!

INGREDIENTS

- 4 potatoes, boiled and grated
- 2-3 zucchini, boiled and grated
- 2-3 carrots, boiled and grated
- ½ cup finely chopped mint
- ½ cup finely chopped parsley
- 1 tomato, grated
- 3 tbsp stale breadcrumbs
- Salt and pepper
- 4 tbsp oil

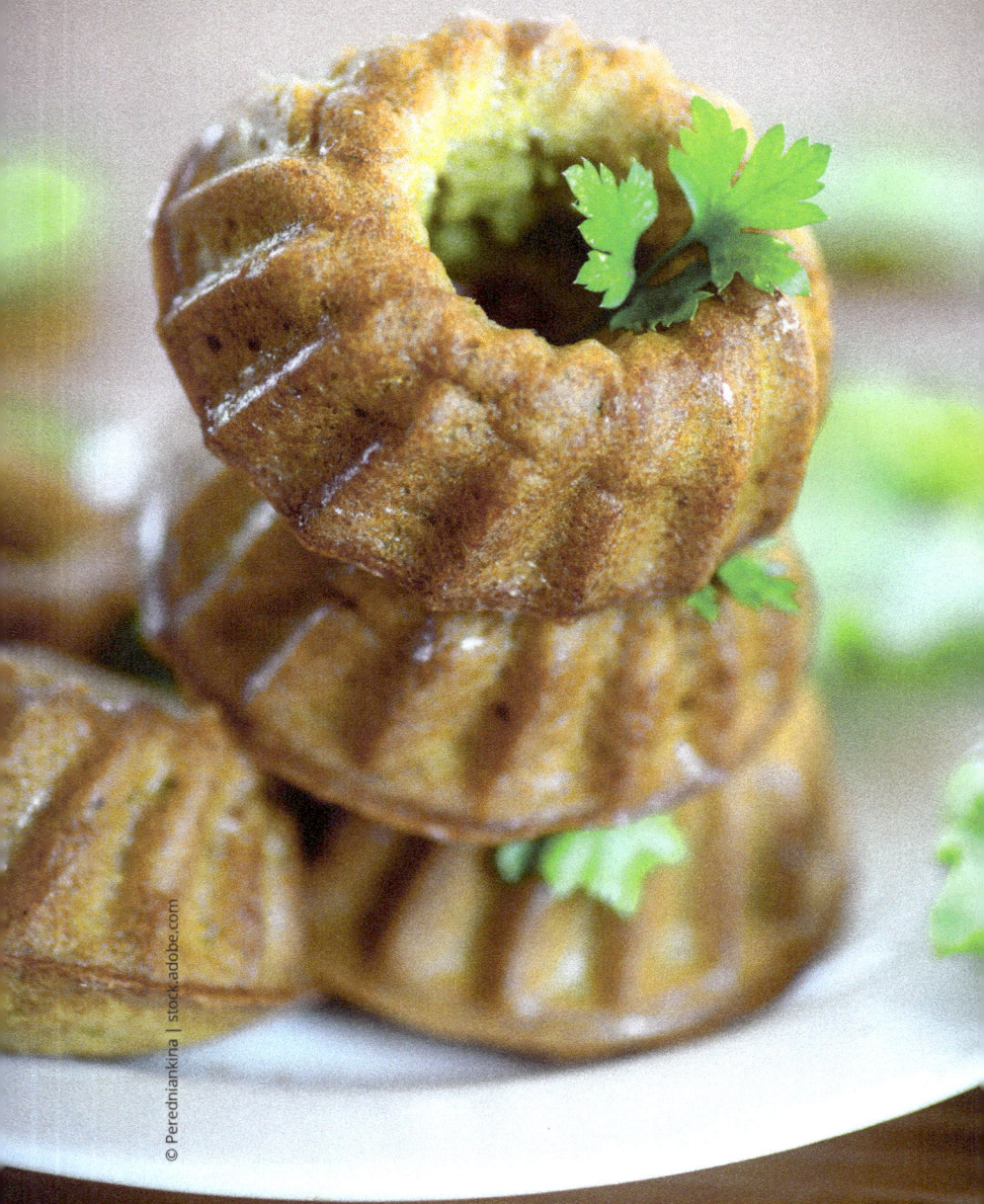

Snack

They will love dairy products

Cheese cupcakes

Preheat the oven to 170-180° C.

In a mixing bowl, I add all the ingredients and stir them to combine well. I divide the mixture into as many small pieces of silicon or paper moulds as I have.

I put them in the oven for 40-45 minutes until they rise and turn a nice golden colour.

This is how we get our children to eat cheese.

As an option, you may add chopped mint in the mixture.

Tip

It is best to serve this without decorating with vegetables and herbs. The kids are not impressed.

It is also best to choose mild, not too salty, cheeses.

INGREDIENTS

- 250 g self-rising flour
- 150 g melted butter
- 150 g Kasseri cheese, grated
- 150 g Gruyère cheese, grated
- 150 g Feta cheese, grated
- 150 g chipolata[1], diced (optional)
- A pinch of pepper
- 3-4 eggs

---

1 *Small thin sausage.*

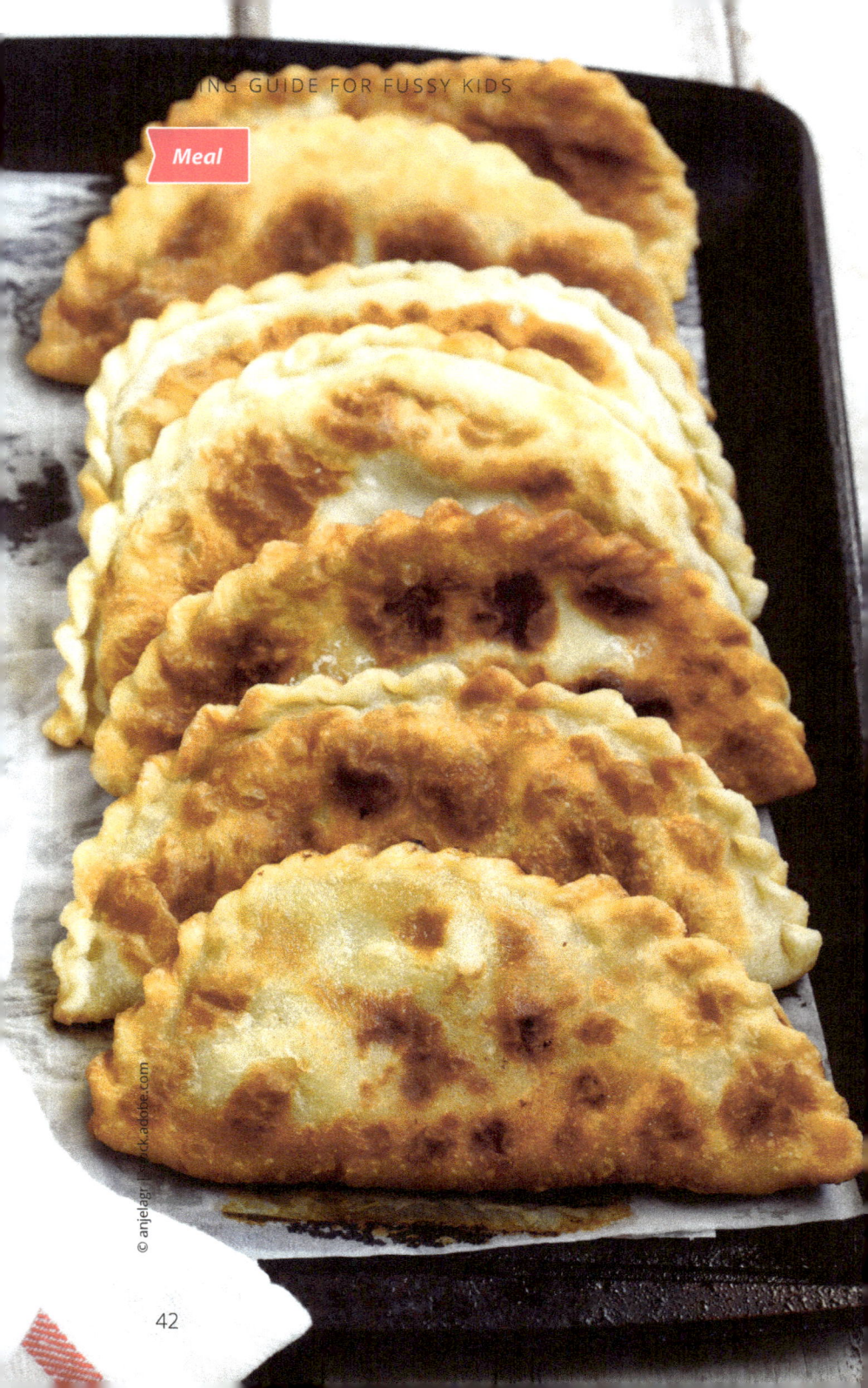

Meal

Perfect for kids all day round

Minced meat pies

I preheat the oven to 180° C.

In a mixing bowl, I combine all the ingredients for the dough, which I knead thoroughly and pat into small balls. In a saucepan, I heat the oil and brown the minced meat and the onion for 3-4 minutes. Then I add the tomato, sugar, salt and pepper, and a glass of water and let that simmer until all the juice is gone. I remove from the heat and let it cool.

With my hands, I pat the dough balls into flat circles, fill each one with one tbsp of the minced meat mixture, and fold the pies closed.

I place them in a greased oven dish, put it in the oven, and bake for 25-30 minutes.

An all-time snack, ideal for everybody, kids especially

INGREDIENTS FOR THE DOUGH

- 500 g self-rising flour
- 200 g soda water

INGREDIENTS FOR THE FILLING

- 100 g sunflower oil
- A pinch of sugar
- A pinch of salt
- 500 g minced meat
- 1 grated onion
- 1 grated tomato
- 3 tbsp oil
- Salt, pepper, sugar

Meal

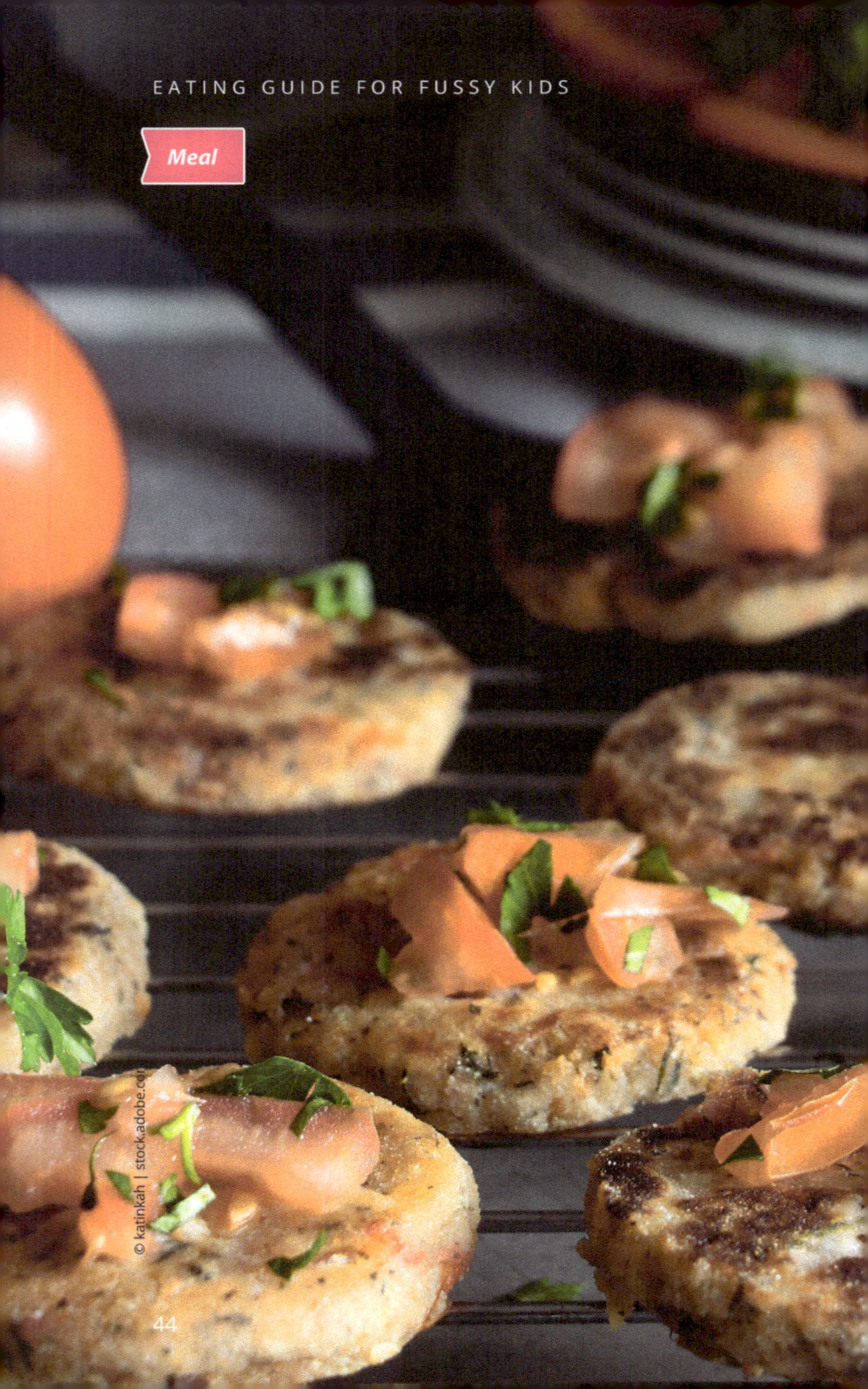

To be served with salad, rice, or whatever the kids fancy

Burgers with roasted tomatoes

I preheat the oven to 180° C.

I cut off the crust of the stale bread, put it in a bowl filled with water, and soak it for half an hour. When I take it out of the water, I wring it as dry as I can. In another clean bowl, I put the minced meat, the bread, the onion, the grated tomato, the egg, parsley, salt, pepper, and oregano, and then I knead.

I grease an oven dish then pat the mixture into burgers and place them in the dish. I roast them for 15 minutes, then flip them over and roast for another 10 minutes. I decorate each burger with a slice of tomato, sprinkle with salt, sugar, and oregano, and roast for another 5 minutes.

Serve with salad, rice or whatever the kids like best.

Tip

Do not decorate with fresh herbs. Usually, the kids don't appreciate them.

INGREDIENTS

- 500 g minced meat, veal
- 250 g stale bread
- 1 onion, grated
- 1 tomato, grated
- 10 tomato slices
- ½ cup finely chopped parsley
- Salt, pepper, oregano, sugar
- 1 egg

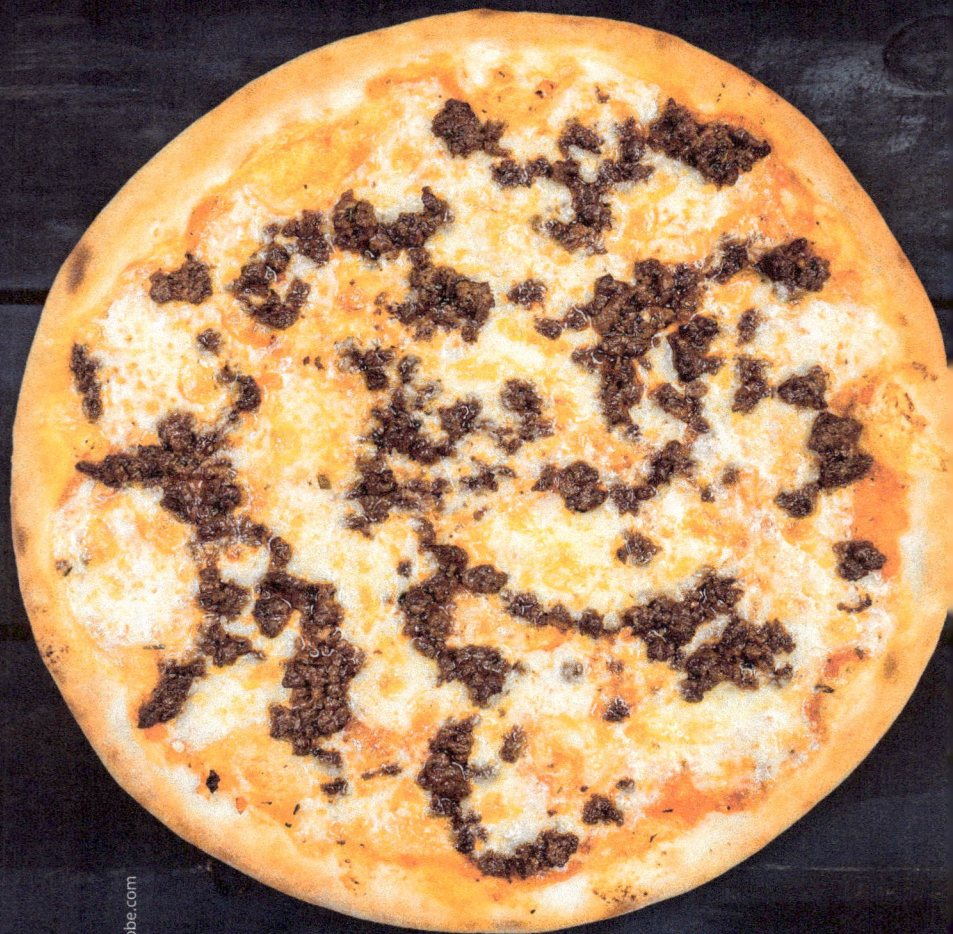

Meal

Perfect for school, the afternoon snack and the party

Kiddies pizza

In a bowl, I put the melted margarine, yoghurt, flour, egg, salt, pepper, and sugar. I knead into soft dough.

In a saucepan, I heat the oil and brown the onion and the meat for 3-4 minutes, then I add the tomato, salt, pepper, sugar, tomato juice, and a glass of water. I let it simmer until the meat is well cooked and the fluid in the saucepan is thick enough.

I pat the dough into small circles, sprinkle them with grated cheese, add a tbsp of the filling right in the centre of each, sprinkle them again with the remaining grated cheese, put them in the oven and bake for 40-45 minutes.

INGREDIENTS FOR THE DOUGH

- 500 g self-rising flour
- 230 g yoghurt
- 230 g margarine
- 1 egg
- Salt, pepper, sugar

INGREDIENTS FOR THE FILLING

- 800 g minced meat, veal
- 2 tomatoes, diced and peeled
- 1 teacup raisins
- 1 water glass of tomato juice
- 1 onion, grated
- 400 g Kasseri cheese, grated
- ½ cup of oil

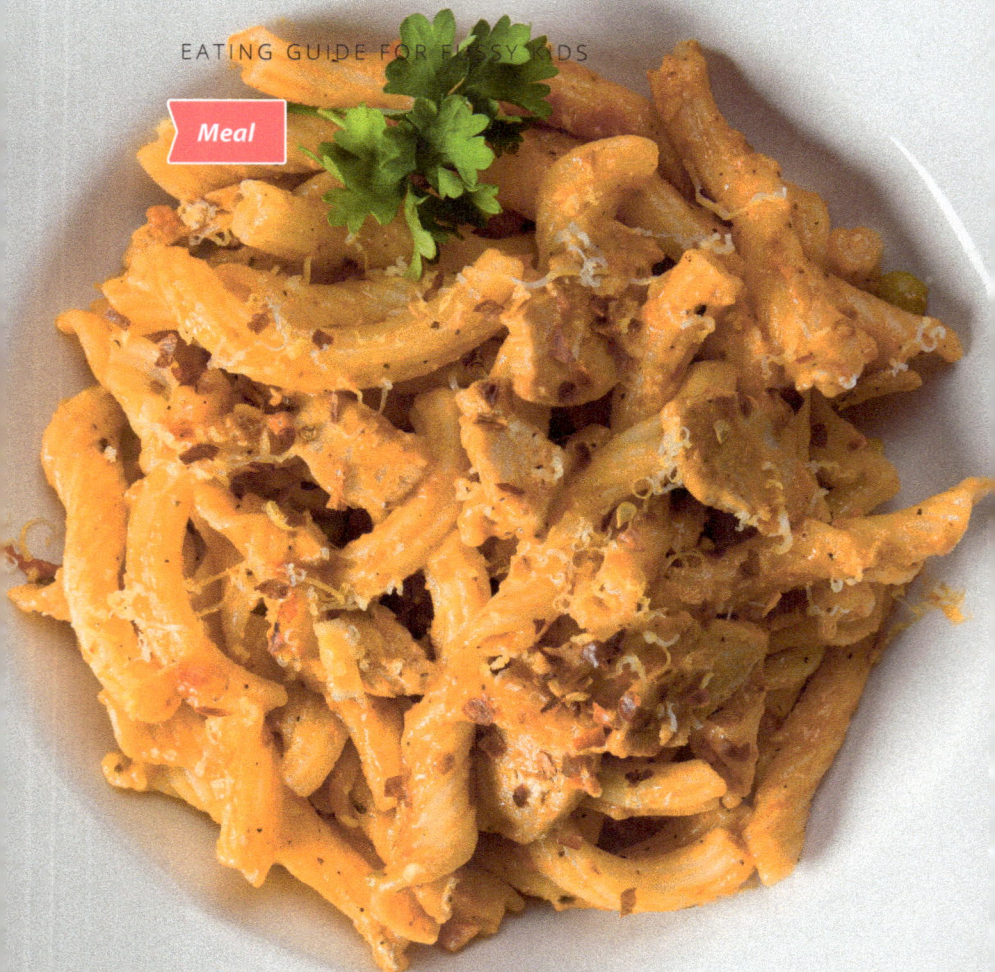

Meal

Tasty bites

Chicken with pasta

I cut the chicken breast in small cubes.

I grease the saucepan with the oil, and when it's hot enough, I brown the chicken and the onion for 4-5 minutes.

I add the tomatoes, salt, pepper, and sugar and bring it to a simmer.

In another saucepan, I prepare the pasta according to the instructions, making sure to remove from heat 3 minutes before the time prescribed.

I strain the pasta and add it to the saucepan with the chicken. I stir all the ingredients to make sure they mix well, allow it to simmer for 2-3 more minutes, and remove from heat.

Sprinkle with the grated cheese and enjoy hot!

Here too, it's better to avoid decorating with parsley!

INGREDIENTS

- 1300 - 1500 g chicken (fillet)
- 1 onion, diced
- 1 kg tomatoes, juiced in the blender
- ½ cup oil
- Salt, pepper, sugar
- 500 g pasta
- 1 cup of grated Kasseri

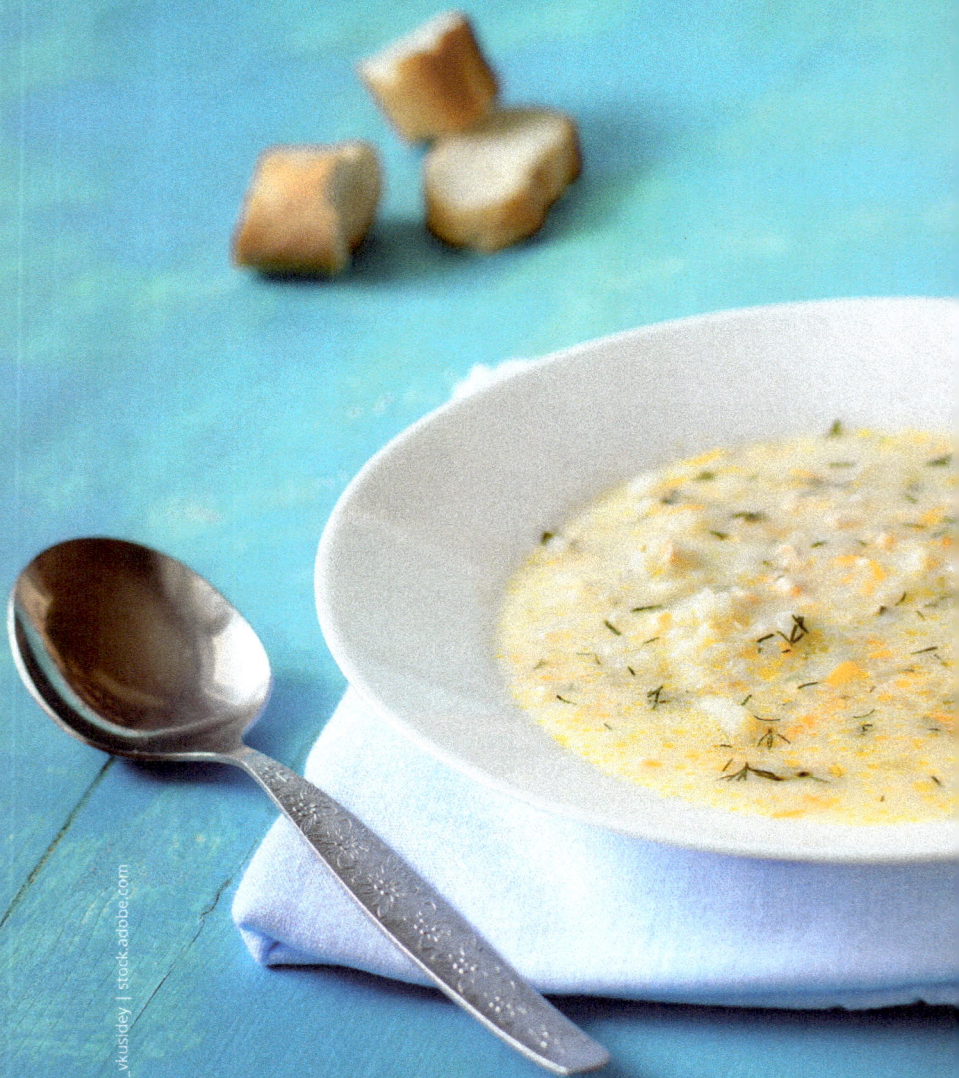

Meal

Starry with pasta

Fish soup

In a saucepan, I put water and bring it to boil. I add the potatoes, carrots, zucchini, celery, lemon juice, salt, and pepper. I let them simmer for 15 to 20 minutes.

Then, I add the fish and let them simmer for another 20 minutes. I remove the saucepan from the heat, and when the fish is cool, I remove the bones very carefully.

I strain the juice from the cocked vegetables and add them to the fish stew. I bring it to a simmer, and when it starts to boil, I add the pasta and let it simmer for another 8 to 10 minutes, stirring constantly. I add the fish cut into small bites and remove the saucepan from the heat.

It is a delicious soup for the whole family.

Variation

To the above ingredients, I add 4 or 5 peeled tomatoes.

INGREDIENTS

- 1 kg fish for soup
- 3-4 small potatoes
- 3-4 carrots, sliced
- 1 onion
- 3-4 zucchini
- 1 teacup pasta for soup
- Celery
- ½ cup lemon juice
- Salt, pepper

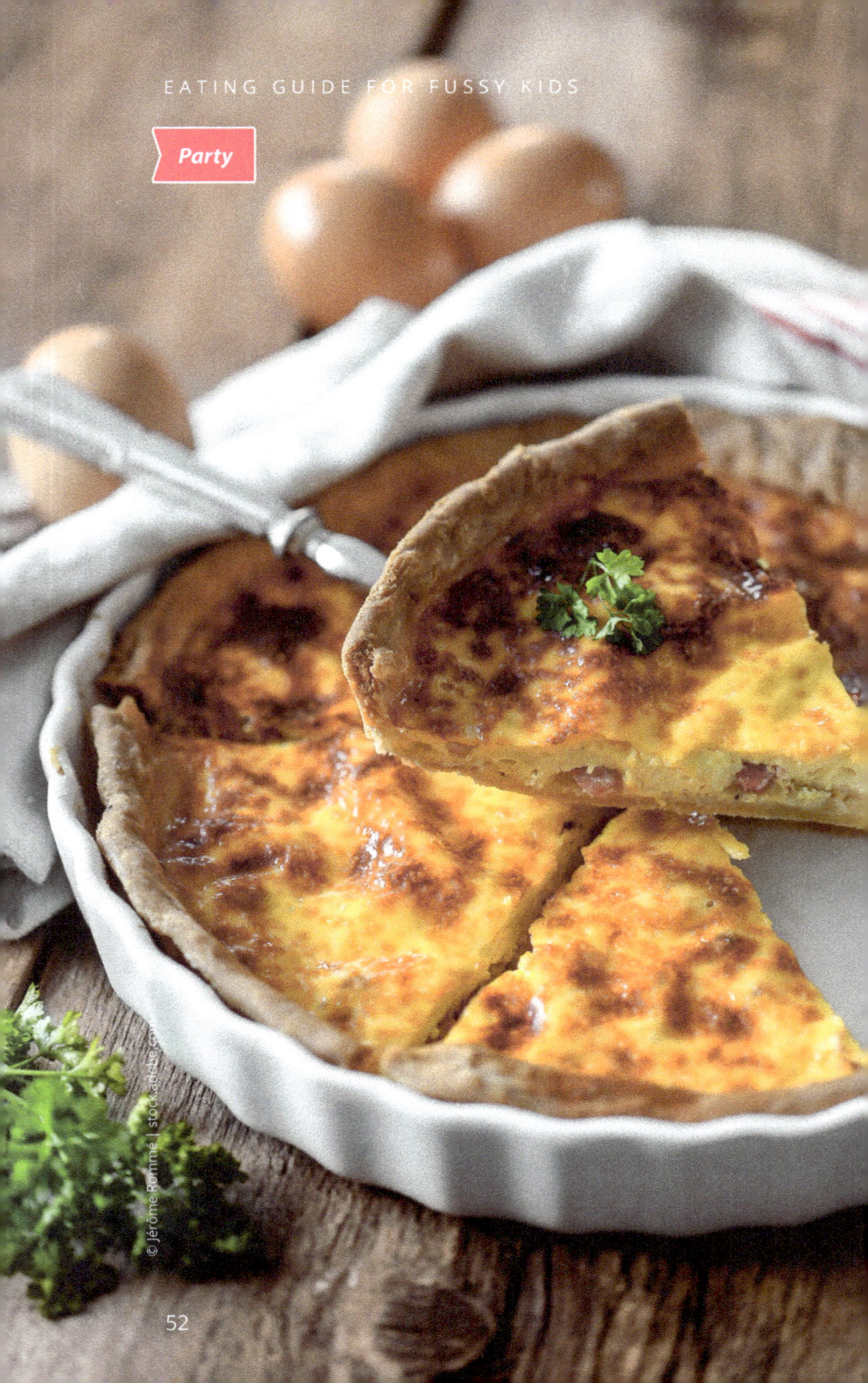

Now, we are having fun!

Savoury Torte

I preheat the oven to 180° C.

In a mixing bowl, I combine all of the ingredients. I may add some finely chopped fresh mint.

I use a cake dish—one with a hole in the middle. I grease it with margarine and line the dish with the first phyllo[1] layer. I oil the phyllo and spread a tablespoon of the mixture on it. I alternate phyllo and mixture (always greasing first each phyllo) until the mix is finished. Then I fold the pastry over, pour the remaining margarine and sprinkle with water. I put the cake dish in the oven and bake for almost 60 minutes. When it's ready, I remove from the oven and let it cool for 5 minutes. Then I upend on a platter.

Tasty and impressive.

---

1 Also filo and filo (phyllo) pastry. A kind of dough that can be stretched into very thin sheets, used in layers to make both sweet and savoury pastries, especially in eastern Mediterranean cooking (Oxford Dictionary).

INGREDIENTS

*   10 layers puffy phyllo (pie crust)

*   150 g melted margarine

*   250 g yoghurt

*   2-3 chipolatas, diced

*   2-3 slices of ham, diced

*   2-3 rashers of bacon, diced

*   2 tbsp cream cheese

*   ½ red pepper and ½ green pepper, both diced

*   300 g grated sweet Kasseri cheese. For grown-ups, you may add blue cheese (see photo)

*   2-3 eggs

53

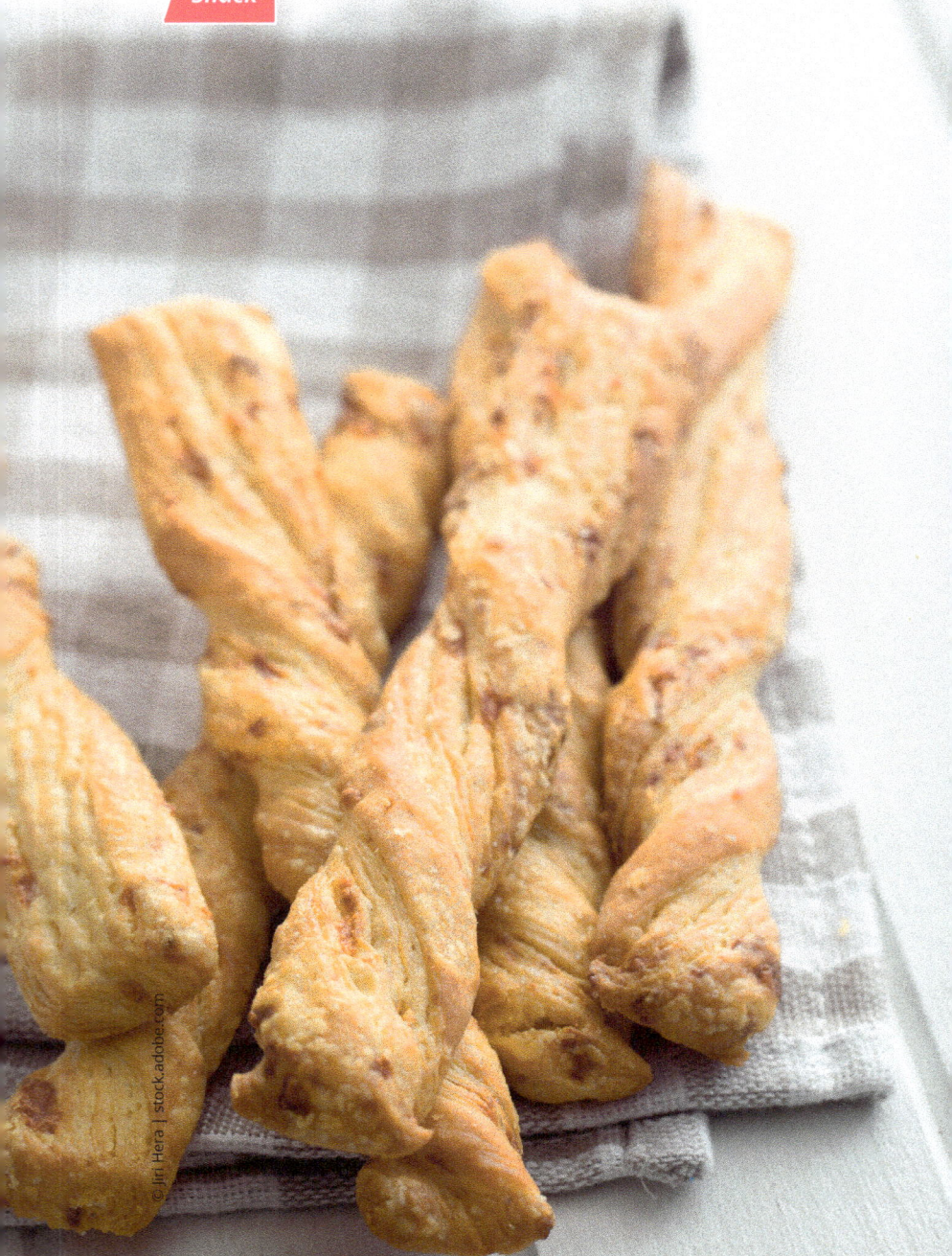

Snack

To be enjoyed at school

Cheesy breadsticks

I preheat the oven to 180° C.

In a mixing bowl, I mix the flour, butter, sugar, the cheese, and milk and knead.

I sprinkle flour on the workbench and pat the dough into breadsticks in any shape I choose.

I put them in a greased oven dish. I brush sparingly with oil and sprinkle the breadsticks with sesame seeds.

I bake for 10-15 minutes.

INGREDIENTS

- 200 g grated cheese (Kasseri)
- 5-6 tbsp melted butter
- 1 cup flour
- 1 pinch of sugar (half a teaspoonful)
- 2 tbsp milk
- ½ cup of sesame seeds
- ½ cup of flour
- ½ cup of oil

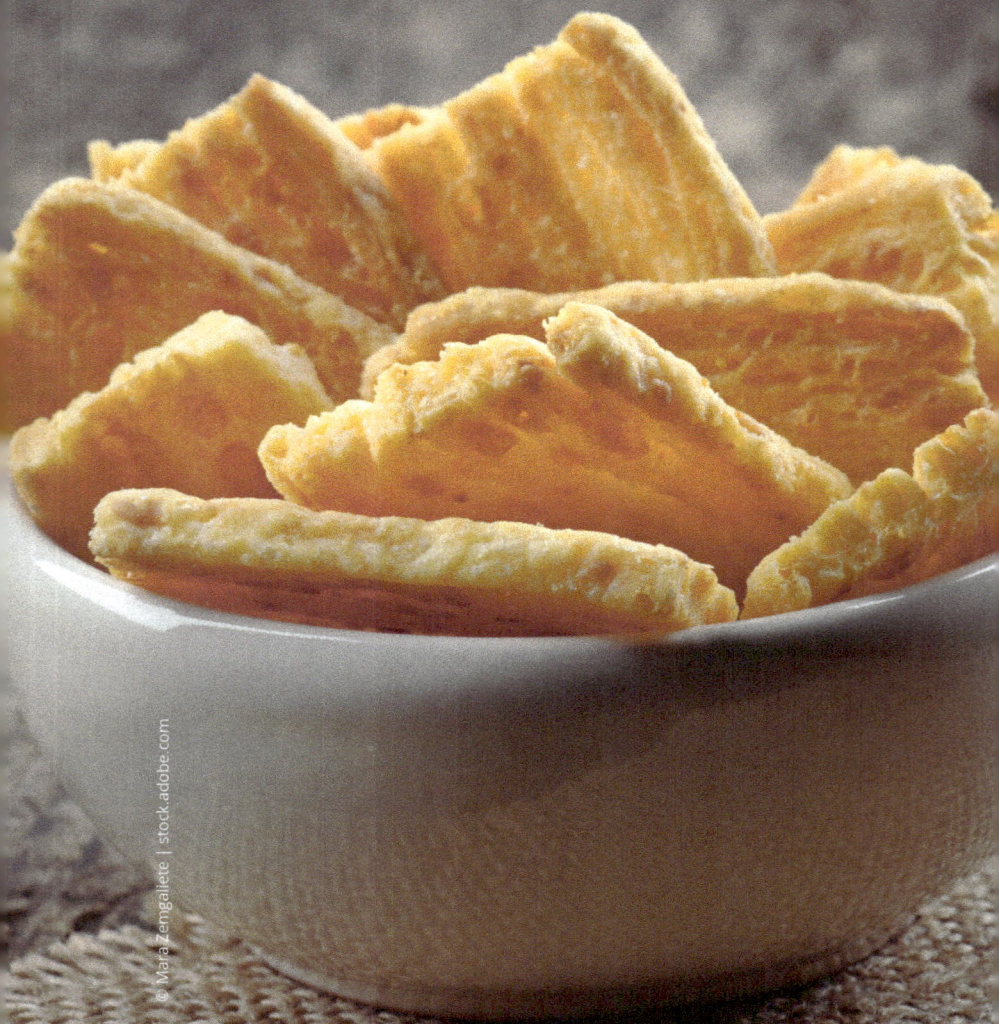

Snack

Savoury biscuits

I preheat the oven to 180° C.

In a bowl, I mix the flour with the baking powder, add the remaining ingredients, and combine them into a soft dough.

Using cookie cutters, I cut the dough in different shapes; then I line the bottom of an oven dish with baking paper on which I place the biscuits.

I bake for 25 minutes.

INGREDIENTS

- 400 g flour
- 60 g pecorino cheese, grated
- 200 g Gruyère, grated
- 200 g cottage cheese, unsalted
- 100 g feta cheese, crushed
- 200 g oil
- 2 eggs
- 1 tsp baking powder
- Leaves of finely chopped mint

Meal

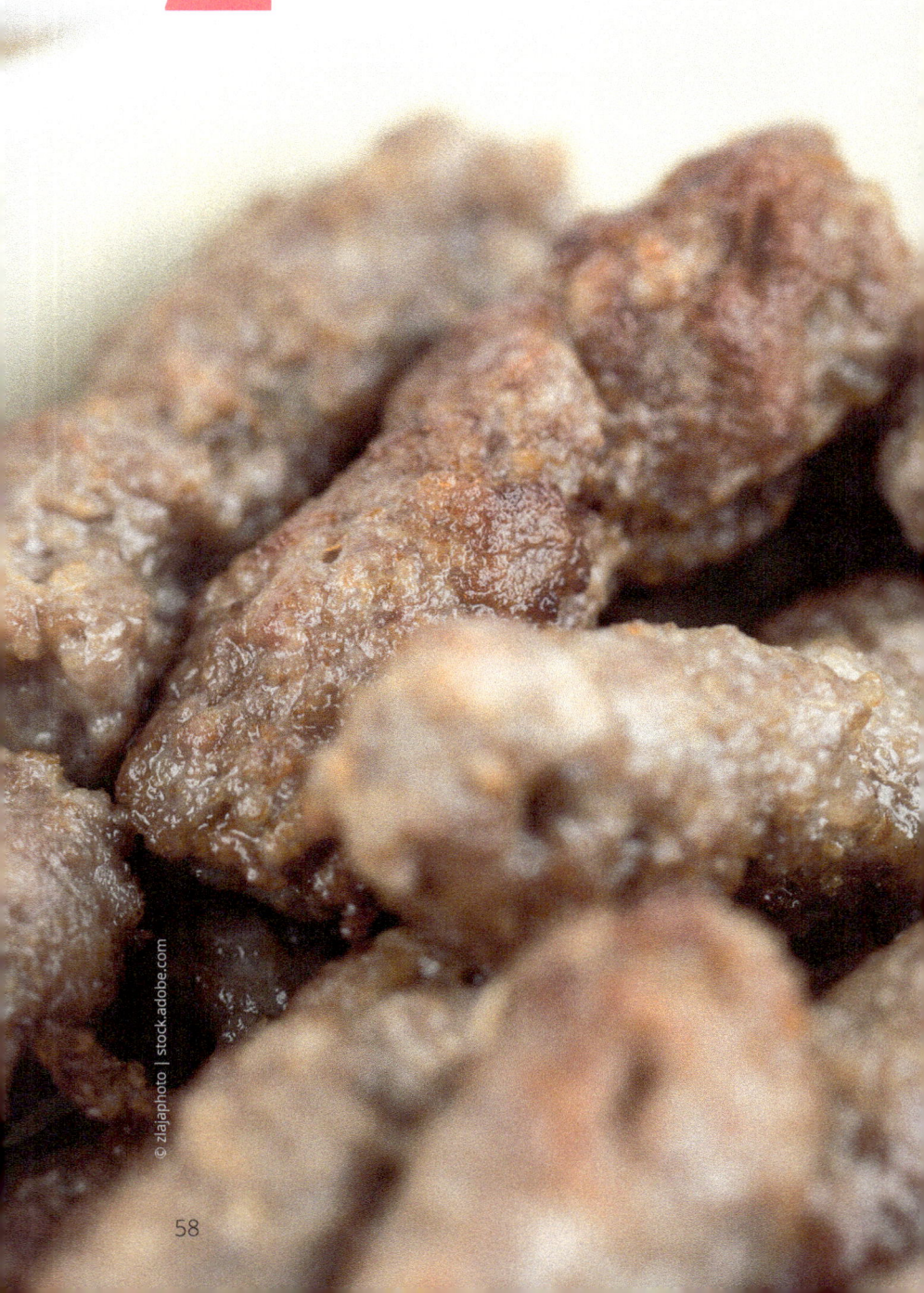

The smaller, the easier it is for the kids to eat

Omelette wraps

I preheat the oven to 180° C.

In a mixing bowl, I put the minced meat, the bread (thoroughly wrung), the onion, the tomato, the salt, pepper, oregano and the finely-chopped parsley. I combine the ingredients and knead them very well. In another bowl, I prepare the egg mix for the omelette: I beat the eggs, and add the tomato and the cheese.

In a non-stick frying pan, I put the oil and pour the egg mixture when the oil gets warm. I fry the omelette for 2-3 minutes then flip it over and turn the heat off. I move the omelette onto a platter. I shape the meat mixture into burgers and put one tbsp of the omelette in the centre of each.

I fold the omelette into the burger and then shape the filled burgers into rolls. I place them on a greased oven dish and grill them for 15 minutes then flip them and grill for another 15 minutes.

Serve hot with French fries.

INGREDIENTS

- 500 g minced meat
- 250 g stale bread soaked in water
- 1 onion, grated
- 1 tomato, grated
- Salt, pepper, oregano, finely chopped parsley

FOR THE OMELETTE

- 3 eggs
- 200 g grated cheese
- 1 tomato, diced
- 2 tbsp oil

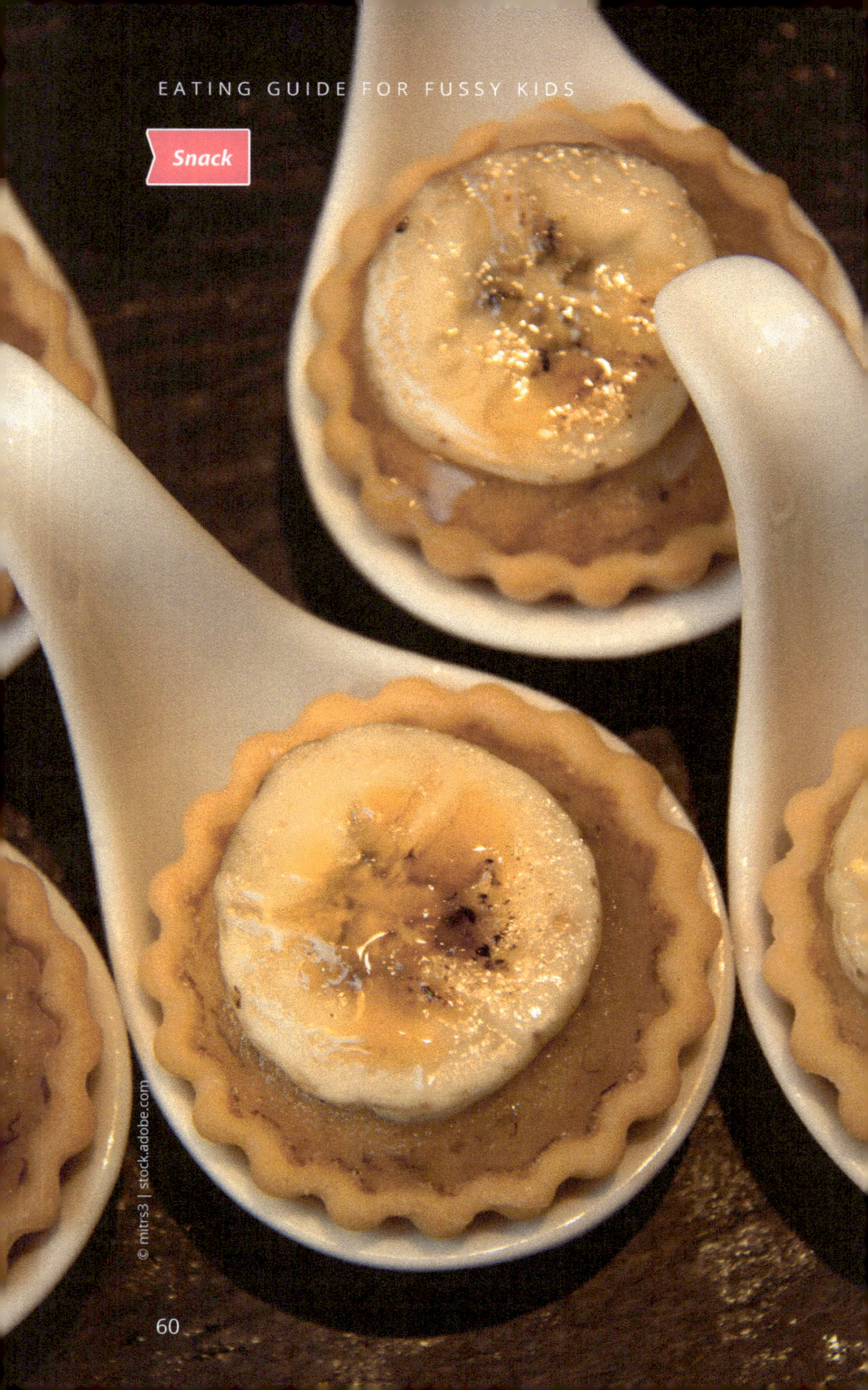

Snack

A different kind of cupcakes

Bananas with chocolate

I preheat the oven to 170° C.

In a mixing bowl, I mix all the ingredients for the cupcakes and knead.

In a dish, I crush the bananas with a fork. In a saucepan, I put the bananas, the sugar, the cinnamon, the hazelnuts, the zest, the juice, and the liqueur then turn the heat on low. I stir and let them cook for 8-10 minutes. I add the chocolate and stir.

I remove from heat.

I pat the dough into small tarts and fill each with a tbsp of the banana mixture.

I put them in an oven dish and bake for approx. 20 minutes.

I let them cool then sprinkle with powdered sugar or decorate with a banana slice and honey.

Variation

You can leave the Grand Marnier out.

INGREDIENTS

- 1 kg bananas
- 1 cup of brown sugar and another cup of crushed hazelnuts
- 1 tbsp cinnamon, powdered
- 1 orange, zest
- ½ cup powdered sugar
- ½ cup lemon juice
- 200 g chocolate, diced
- 3 tsp Grand Marnier

FOR THE CUPCAKES

- 4 cups of flour
- ½ cup milk and ½ cup oil
- ½ tsp baking powder
- ½ tsp sugar and ½ tsp salt

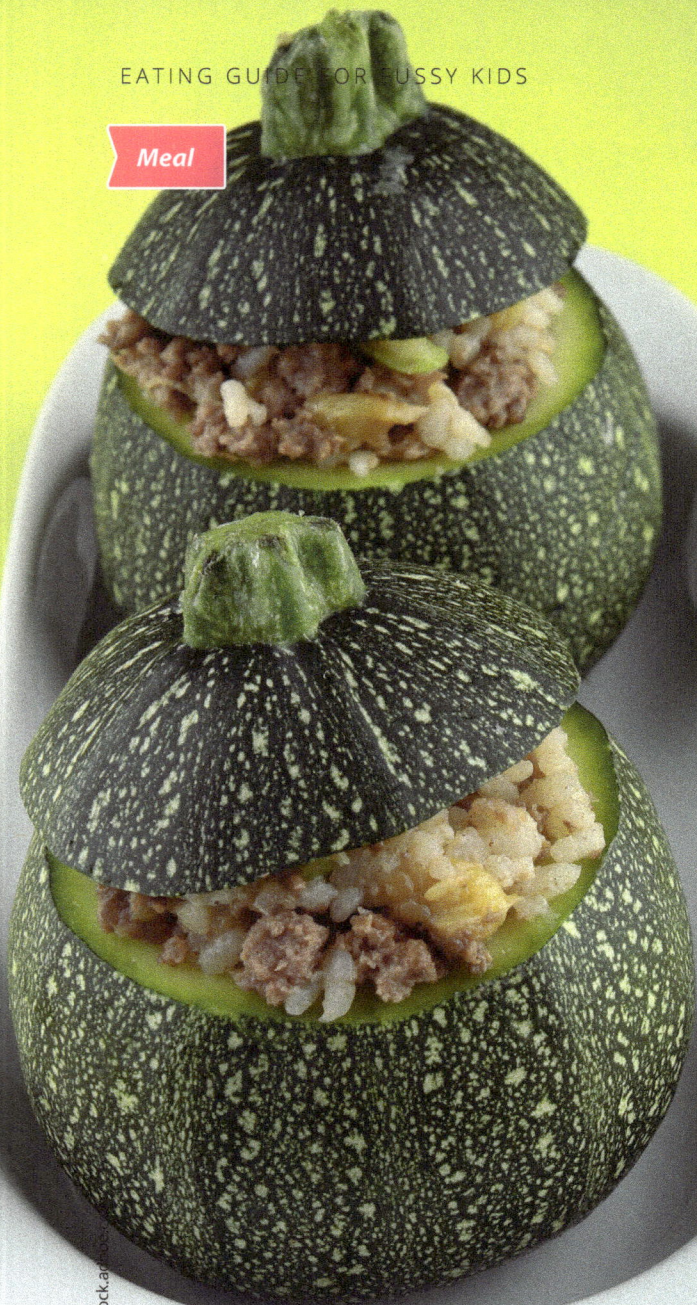

Meal

62

Stuffed zucchini

Barrels

I wash the zucchini, cut their tops off, and core them carefully with a spoon.

I heat the oil in a pan, brown the onion and the minced meat for 2-3 minutes, then add the tomato juice, salt, pepper, sugar, and parsley plus 1 cup of water. I bring it to a simmer and add the rice.

I stir regularly and bring to a simmer again until the sauce in the pan thickens. I remove from the heat and let it cool.

I fill each zucchini and cover them with their tops. I place them in a wide saucepan: add a cup of water, the oil and the flesh of the zucchini, finely chopped.

I season and bring to a simmer until the zucchini is cooked.

The kids appreciate the round, barrel-like shape of the zucchini.

INGREDIENTS

- 10 round zucchini
- 500 g minced meat
- 1 onion, grated
- 1 glass tomato juice
- ½ cup oil
- ½ bunch finely chopped parsley
- Salt, pepper, sugar
- ½ cup rice
- ½ cup oil

Snack - Side dish

We may sprinkle with sesame before baking

Walnut buns

I preheat the oven to 200° C.

In a mixing bowl, I put the flour, the oil, sugar, the salt, and the beer. I knead the mixture thoroughly in a dough and then pat it into small circles. I place a tbsp of walnuts in the centre of each, fold closed, and reshape them into little buns.

I line a baking dish with baking paper and place the buns. I cover them with cling film and let them rise for 30 minutes. Then I take it off and bake for 40-45 minutes.

Variation

Alternatively, I may use finely diced sun-dried tomatoes instead of walnuts.

INGREDIENTS

- 1 small tin of beer[1] (200 g)
- 500 g self-rising flour
- 1 tbsp oil
- 1 tbsp sugar
- 1 tsp salt
- 200 g crushed walnuts

----

1 *Beer for the yeast.*

Meal

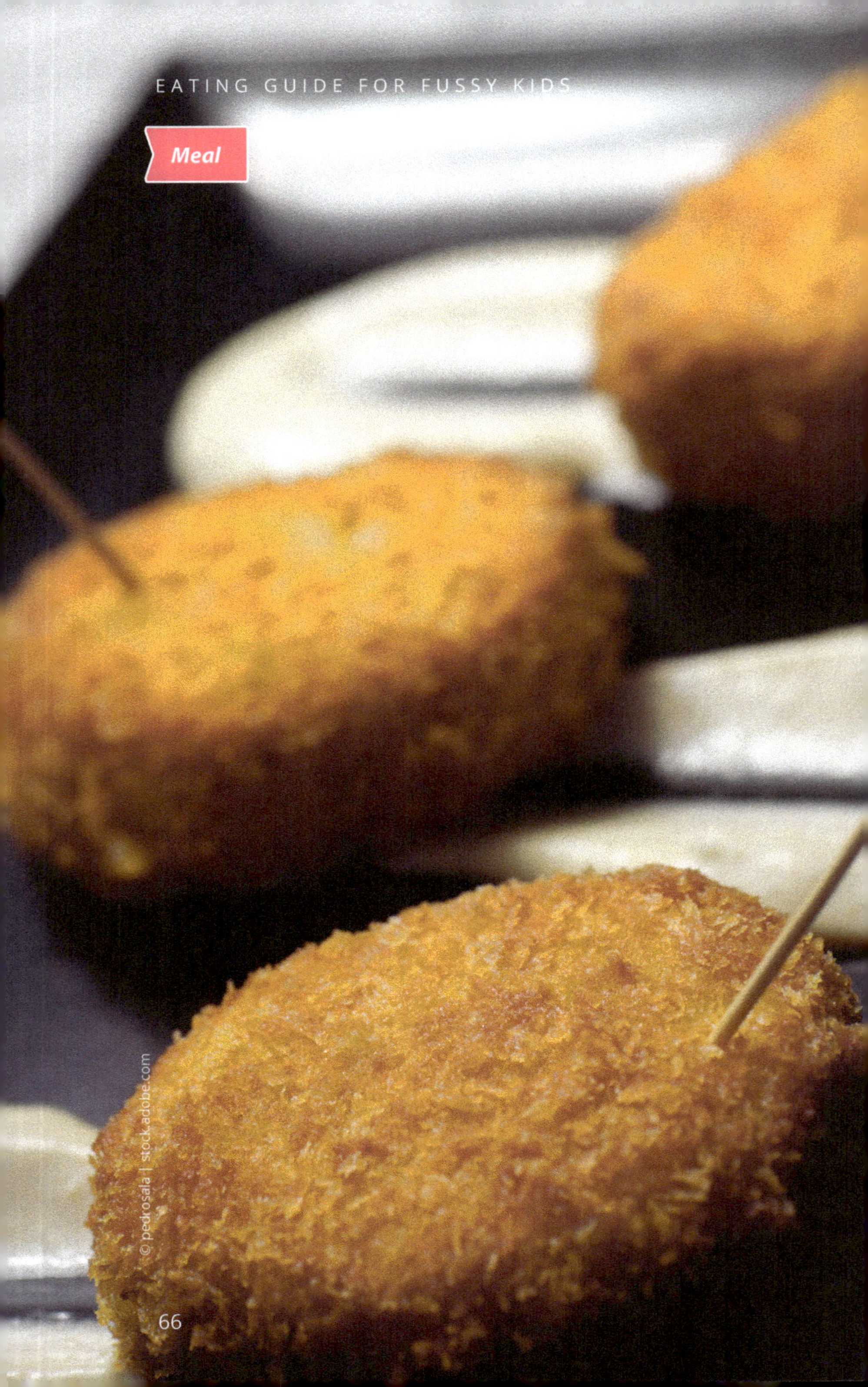

Can be used as a snack or school lunch

Chicken croquet

In a mixing bowl, I combine the minced chicken, onion, parsley, eggs, breadcrumbs, salt, pepper and the oil. I knead the mixture and cover it with cling film, then put it in the fridge for an hour.

In the meantime, I sprinkle one platter with the flour and another with the breadcrumbs, and I beat the eggs with the oil separately.

I then heat the oil, pat the chicken mixture into croquettes, and roll them in the flour, then the egg, then the breadcrumbs, and fry them.

I fry them carefully, one at a time, and remove them subsequently with a slotted spoon.

Serve hot or cold! Ideal snack for school!

INGREDIENTS

- 1 kg chicken minced meat
- ½ bunch finely chopped parsley
- 1 onion, grated
- 2 eggs
- 200 g breadcrumbs
- Salt, pepper
- ½ cup oil

FOR THE BREADING

- 400 g flour
- 2-3 eggs
- 300 g breadcrumbs
- 3-4 tbsp oil

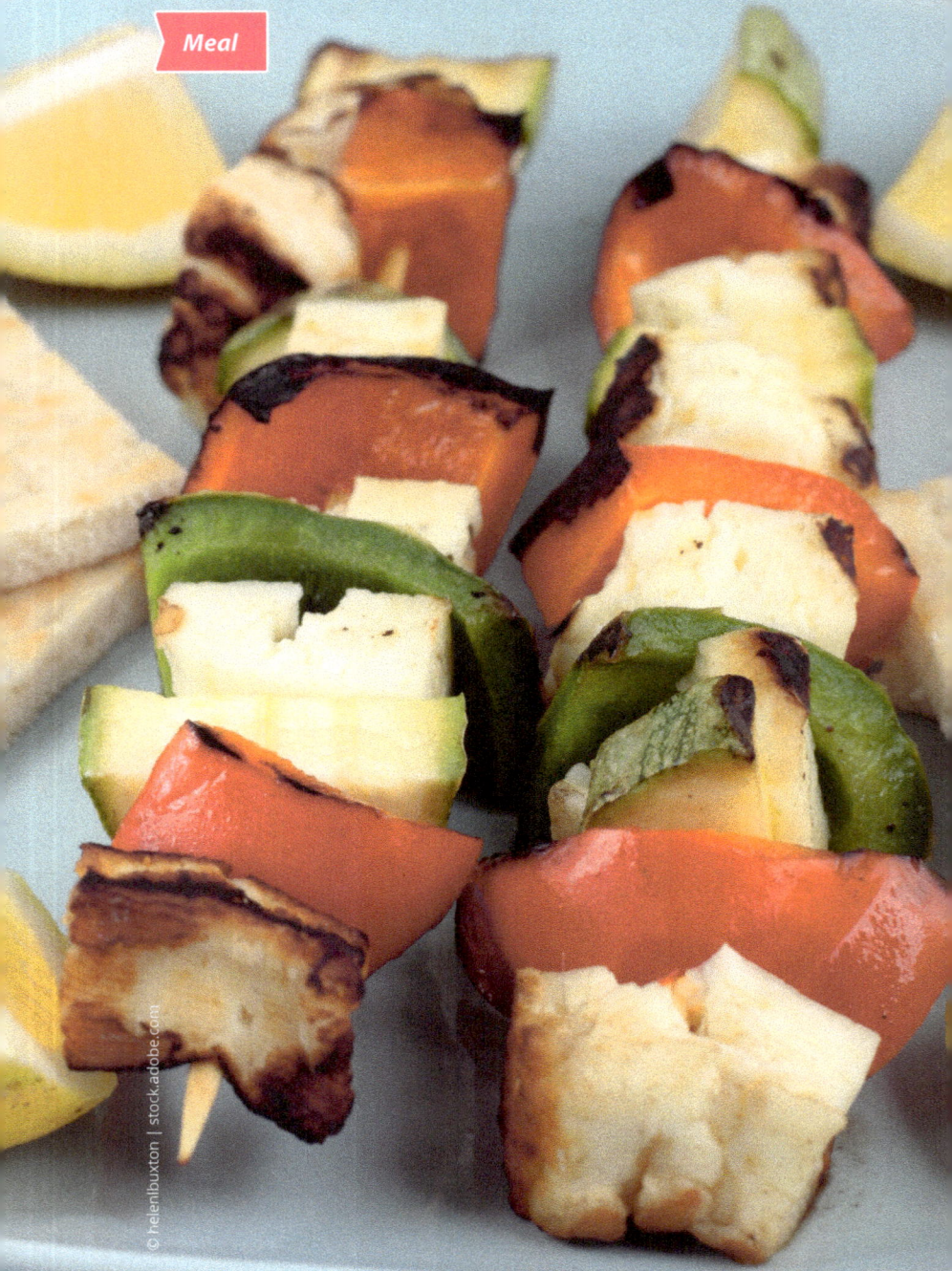

Meal

With feta, ham and cherry tomatoes

Souvlaki[1]

In a bowl, I place the feta with all the herbs, and put it aside for 30 minutes.

Then I take one skewer at a time, and, alternately, I thread a cherry tomato, a cube of feta, a cherry tomato, a cube of ham and so on.

I have prepared French fries, which I serve with the souvlaki! Delicious for the kids!

Variations

On the skewer, you may use any combination of vegetables and cheeses you wish.

INGREDIENTS

- 20 small cubes feta cheese, the size of a walnut
- 20 small cubes ham, the size of a walnut
- 20 cherry tomatoes, whole
- ½ bunch freshly and finely chopped oregano
- ½ cup oil
- 1 tbsp fresh thyme
- Skewers

---

1 *A Greek dish of pieces of meat grilled on a skewer: a generous plate of souvlaki, i.e., souvlakia in pitta [pitta: flat, hollow, slightly leavened bread which can be split open to hold a filling] (Oxford Dictionary).*

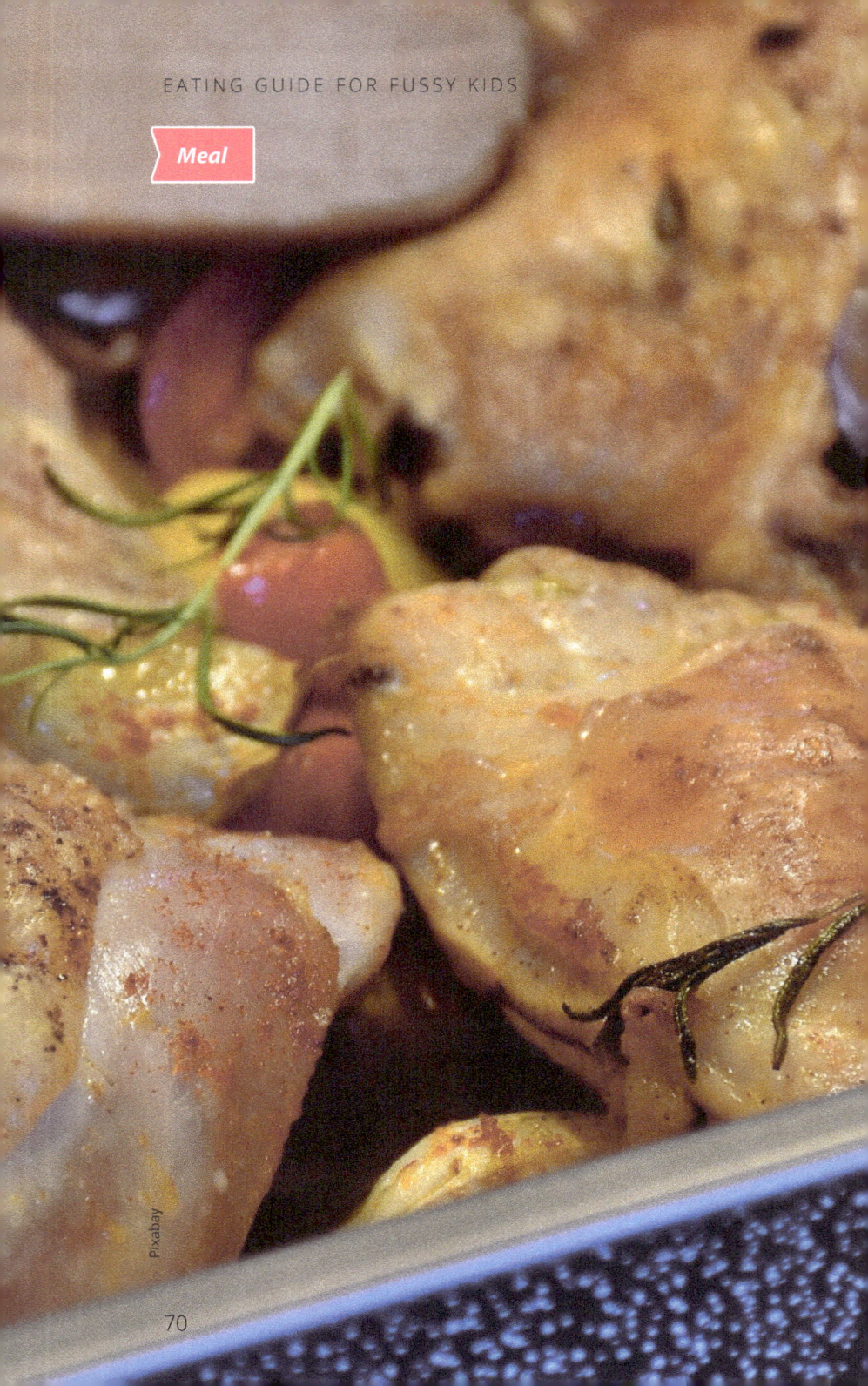

Meal

With cherry tomatoes

Roast chicken

I preheat the oven to 180° C.

I wash and cut the chicken in portions. In a mixing bowl, I put the potatoes, season them, add the cherry tomatoes, the flesh and the zest of the oranges, the oil, salt, pepper, and oregano and mix them well. In an oven dish, I place the chicken and the other ingredients, add 2 cups of water, cover with foil, and bake for 50-55 minutes. I might have to add some water to avoid making it too dry.

I take away the foil and bake for another 10 minutes until it gets a nice golden brown colour.

INGREDIENTS

- 1 chicken, about 1200-1500 g

- 1 kg baby potatoes

- 500 g cherry tomatoes

- 2-3 oranges

- ½ cup oil

- ½ cup lemon juice

- Salt, pepper, oregano

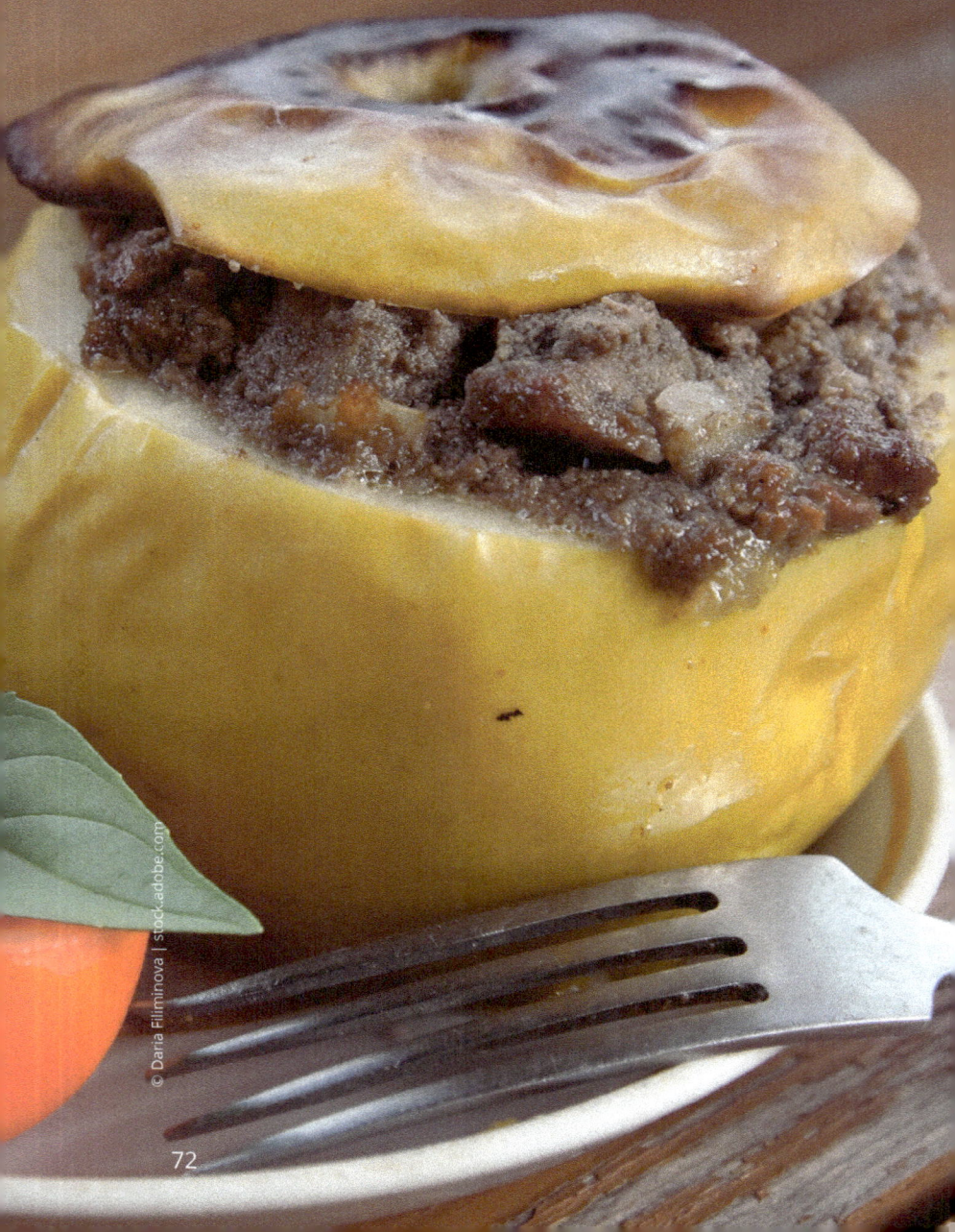

Meal

© Daria Filiminova | stock-adobe.com

You wouldn't believe the taste!

Stuffed apples with minced meat

I core the apples (like I co the stuffed tomatoes) and sprinkle them with the lemon juice to preserve their white colour.

I heat the oil in a saucepan, and I brown the onion and the minced meat for 4-5 minutes. I add the tomatoes and the toma-to juice and the salt and pepper and bring it to a simmer. When the meat is ready, I remove from the heat and let it cool. Then I fill the apples and cover each with its top.

I place all the filled apples in a wide saucepan. I add the flesh of the apples, the oil, and the tomato paste diluted in one cup of water. I bring it to a simmer and shake the saucepan in reg-ular intervals to keep the food from sticking to the bottom.

You can also bake them in the oven like the classically stuffed tomatoes.

INGREDIENTS

- 10-12 apples
- 500 g minced meat
- ½ cup oil
- 1 glass tomato juice
- 1 tbsp tomato paste
- 2 whole tomatoes, peeled
- Salt, pepper
- 1 tbsp lemon juice
- 1 onion, diced
- ½ cup oil

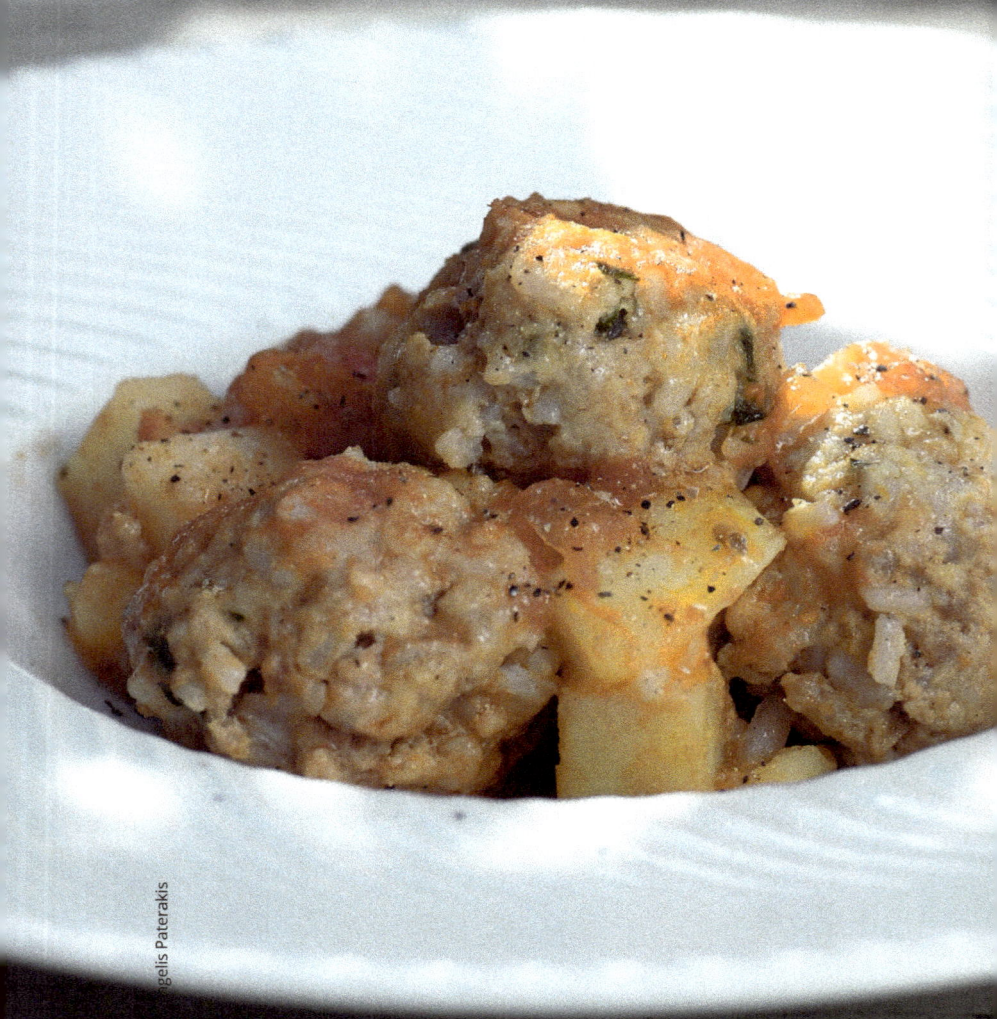

Meal

Kids love them!

Granny's meatballs

In a mixing bowl, I put the meat, onion, rice, egg, the grated tomato, salt, and pepper.

I knead thoroughly and shape the mixture in balls the size of a walnut. I spread the flour on a platter and roll the balls in it. In a big saucepan, I bring water to boil and drop the diced potatoes, the lemon juice, the oil, the diced tomatoes, salt, and let the potatoes simmer for 10-15 minutes. Then I add the meatballs and let it simmer until the meat is done and the sauce thickens.

A healthy meal for the kids.

INGREDIENTS

- 500 g minced meat (veal)
- 200 g rice
- 1 egg
- 1 tomato, grated
- 1 onion, grated
- 1 small bunch of finely chopped parsley
- Salt, pepper
- ½ cup of oil
- ½ cup of lemon juice
- 3-4 potatoes, diced
- 2-3 tomatoes, diced
- Flour and ½ cup of oil

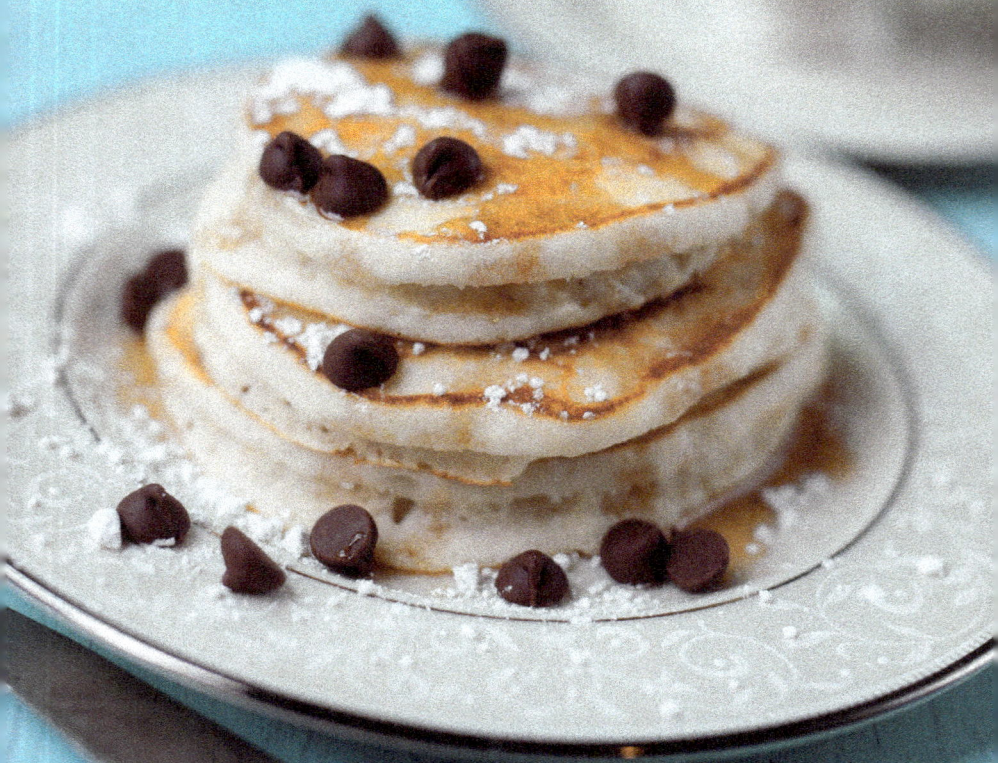

Pure delight!

Pancakes with chocolate flakes

In a bowl, I mix the flour with the baking powder.

I add the eggs, sugar, milk, salt, and the lemon zest. I combine them in a smooth batter. I heat the oil in the frying pan and fry the batter with the help of a spoon, one tbsp at a time.

I flip them over and then remove from the heat. I place the pancakes on a platter and decorate with chocolate flakes.

Variations

Alternatively, you may sprinkle the pancakes with chocolate syrup, caramel, honey, jam, powdered sugar, and whatever catches your fancy!

INGREDIENTS

- 4 eggs
- ½ cup of sugar
- 1 cup of milk
- 2 cups of all-purpose flour
- 1 tbsp baking powder
- A pinch of salt
- Lemon zest
- 200 g chocolate flakes
- Frying oil

Meal

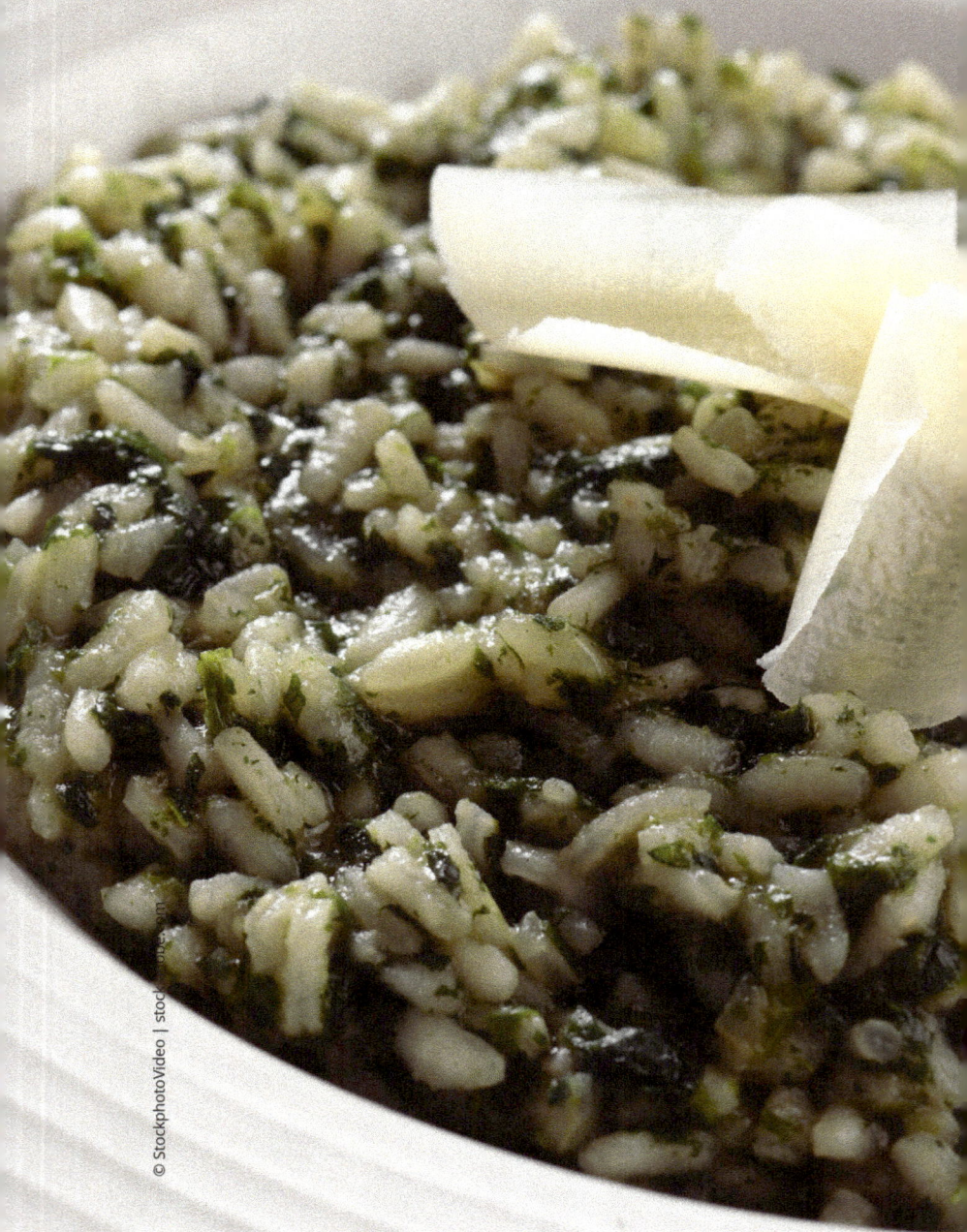

The underrated...

Spinach with rice

I wash and finely chop the spinach and let it dry.

I heat the oil in a saucepan and brown the spring onions for 3-4 minutes. I add the spinach, the rice, salt and pepper, and the tomato. I also add a glass of warm water and bring to a simmer, often stirring so that the rice doesn't stick to the bottom. When the rice is done, I add the dill, the lemon juice, and the zest and let it simmer for another 2-3 minutes. Then I remove from the heat.

The water I add to the rice has to be warm so that it will not get mushy.

As a variation, I may add the flesh of an orange to the food.

Tips

First, kids love lemon, and second, they like cheese. Therefore, you can serve the spinach and rice with some grated cheese, feta or parmesan.

INGREDIENTS

* 1 kg spinach
* ½ cup rice
* ½ cup oil
* ½ bunch of finely chopped dill
* 7-8 spring onions, thinly sliced
* 1 whole tomato, peeled
* 2 tbsp lemon juice
* Salt, pepper
* Lemon zest

SERVING PORTION

* You may serve the spinach with rice in a bowl, like you serve pilaf, in the form of a small hill.

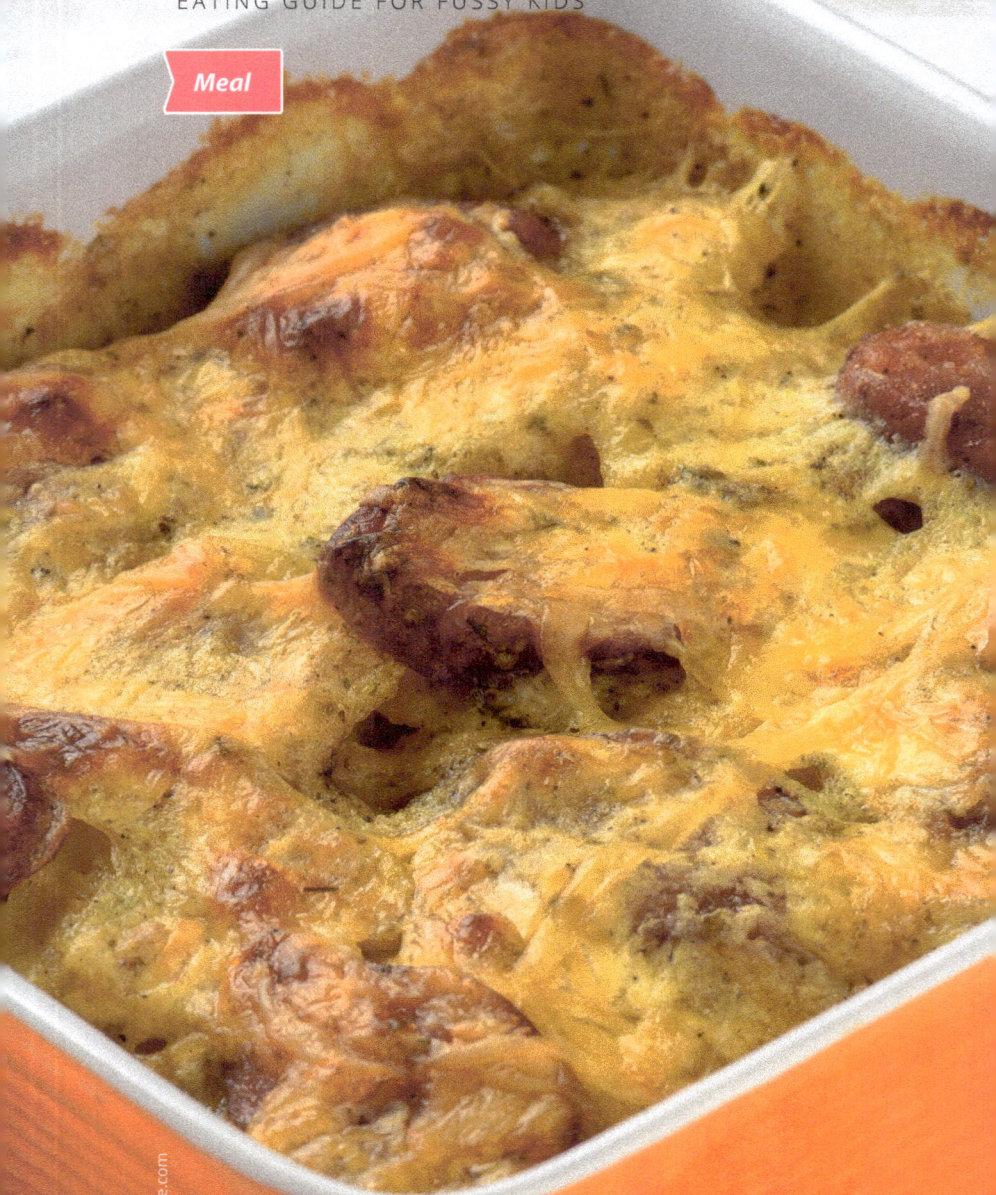

Meal

....

The chipolatas are optional

....

Baby potatoes with feta cheese

In a frying pan, I heat the oil and brown the onion and add the sausages cut in two, the potatoes, and the cherry tomatoes whole. I add the salt, cinnamon, and sugar, and a glass of warm water. I bring to a simmer until the juice thickens.

When it is ready, I add feta, let it simmer for 2-3 more minutes, and remove from the heat.

Alternatively, instead of feta, I may use Kasseri cheese cut in cubes the size of walnuts.

Variation

We may use yellow cheeses or a mixture of yellow cheeses and feta. We may also cook the meal in a Pyrex dish in the oven (see picture).

INGREDIENTS

- 1 kg of baby potatoes, whole
- 10-12 chipolatas
- 10-12 cherry tomatoes, whole
- ½ cup of oil
- Salt, cinnamon, sugar
- 1 onion, diced
- 200 g feta cheese, crushed

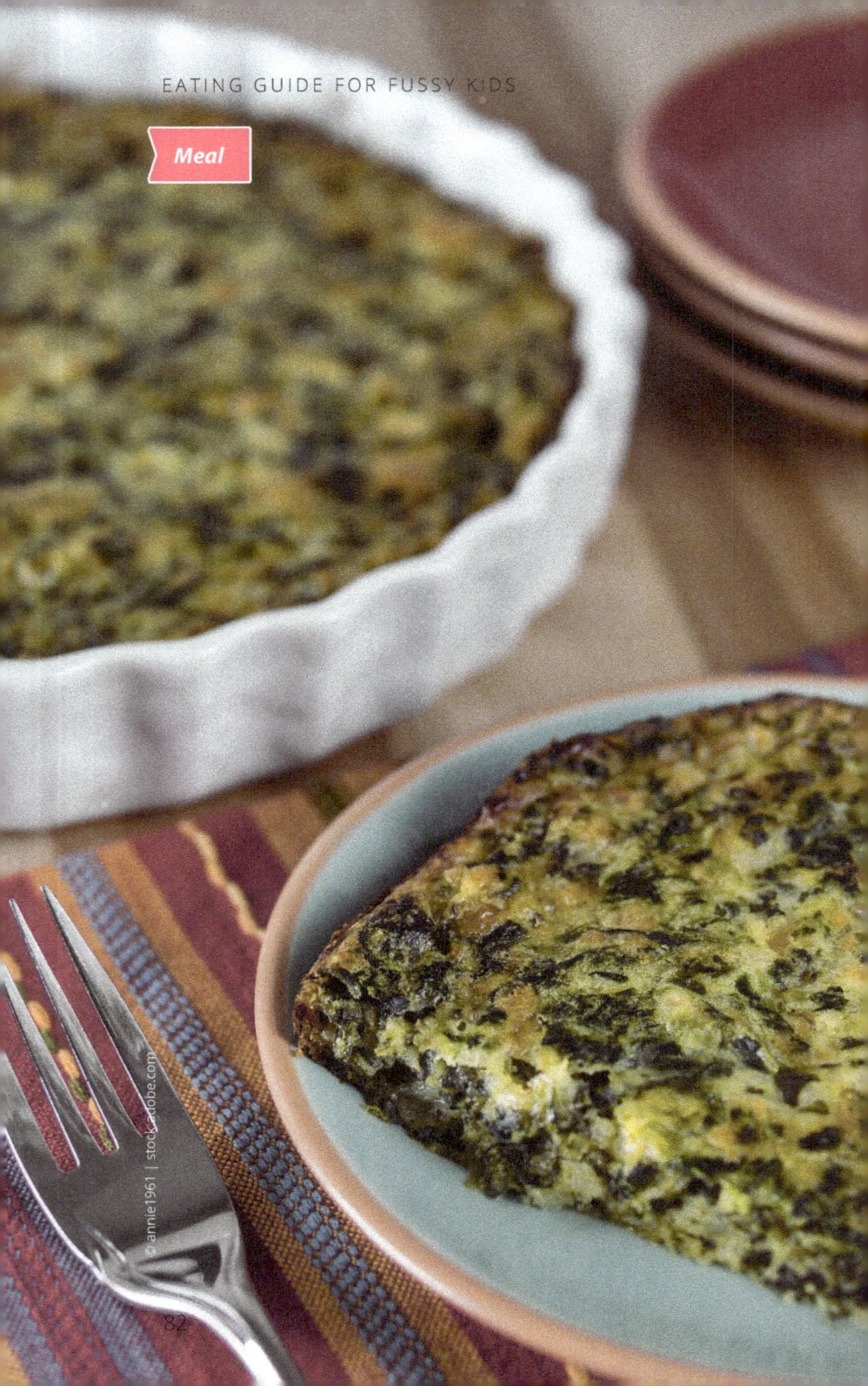

Meal

May also be cooked and served in individual bowls

Spinach with cheeses

I preheat the oven to 180° C.

I wash the spinach thoroughly and let it dry. I put water in a saucepan and bring it to a boil. Then add the spinach and let it boil for 2-3 minutes. I then put it in a colander and strain it.

I grease an oven dish and spread the spinach evenly.

In a mixing bowl, I put the eggs, the cheeses, and ham; I mix them well and spread this mixture on top of the spinach. As a final layer, I add the breadcrumbs.

I put it in the oven and bake for 20-25 minutes.

INGREDIENTS

* 1.5 kg spinach
* 400 g yellow kinds of cheese, grated
* 3 eggs
* 4 slices of ham, diced
* 1 tbsp butter
* 4 tbsp dry breadcrumbs

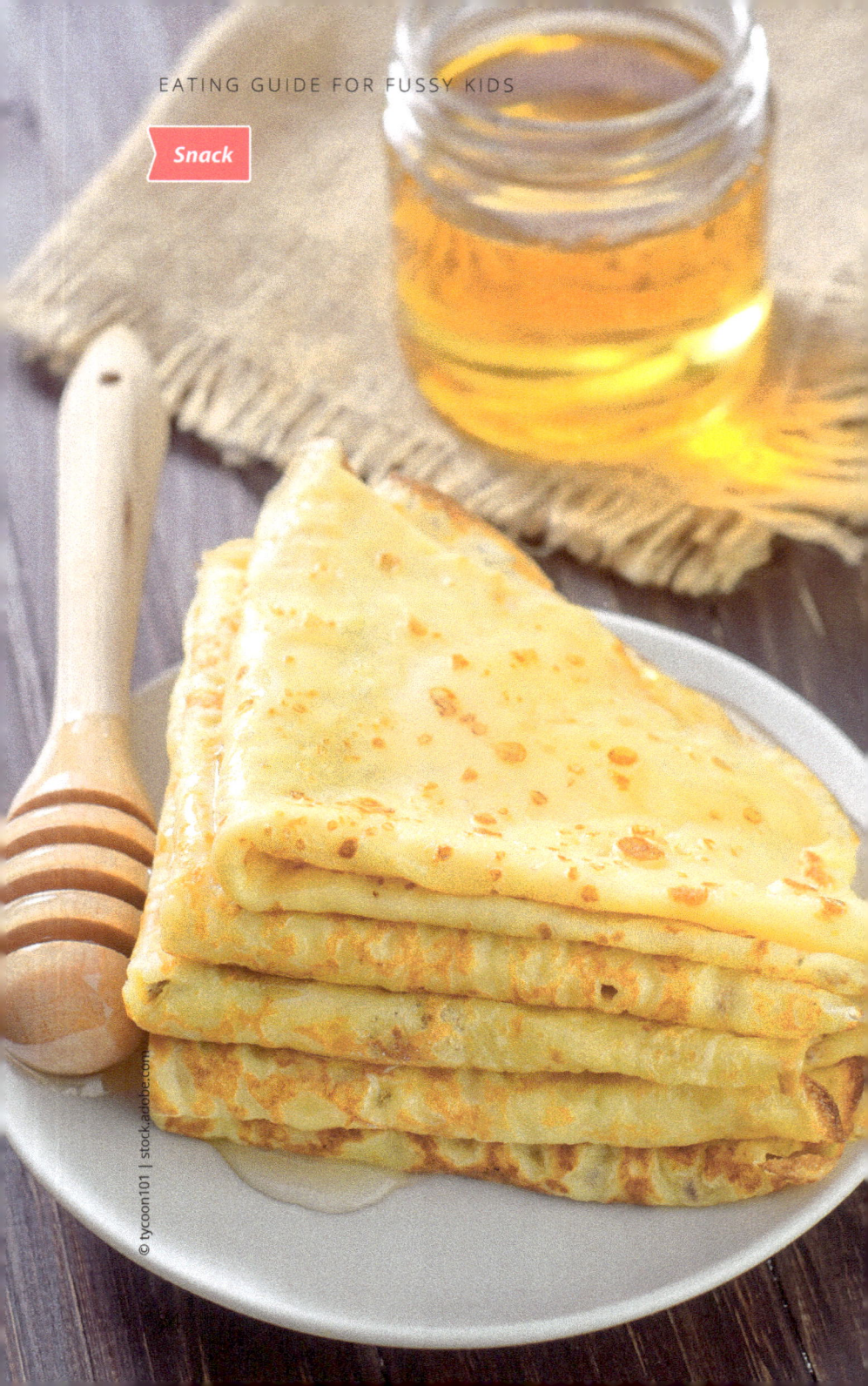

Snack

Also cooked and served in individual portions like a pancake

Omelette with honey

In a mixing bowl, I put the flour. I beat the eggs and add the milk, salt, pepper and paprika. I mix them all well into a smooth batter.

I heat the oil in the frying pan and fry the batter in spoonfuls.

I flip over each omelette and then place them on a platter and sprinkle them with honey, lemon zest and the crushed hazelnuts.

It is a nice, wholesome meal for the kids.

INGREDIENTS

- 6 eggs
- 2 tbsp all-purpose flour
- 4 tbsp milk
- Salt, pepper, sweet paprika
- Honey
- Crushed hazelnuts - Lemon zest
- Frying oil

Section 3

Dad shares his own experience.

From Chef Eirini Togia he gathered inspiration; the imagination, the dishes, and the tricks are all his.

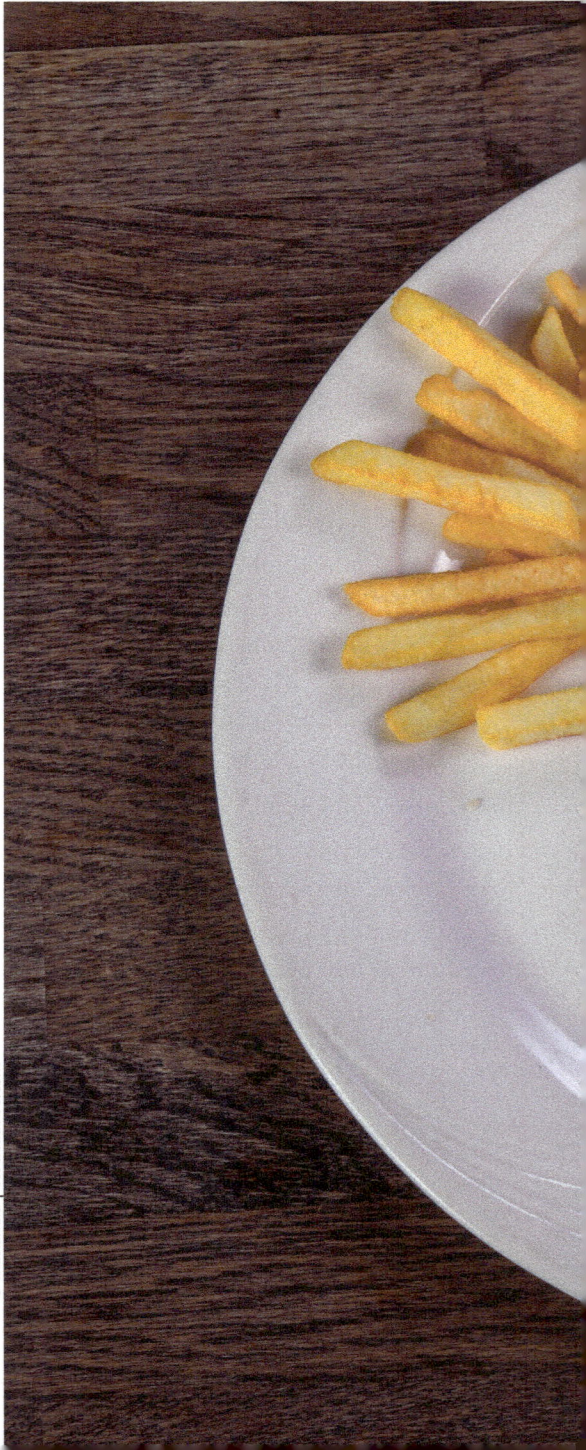

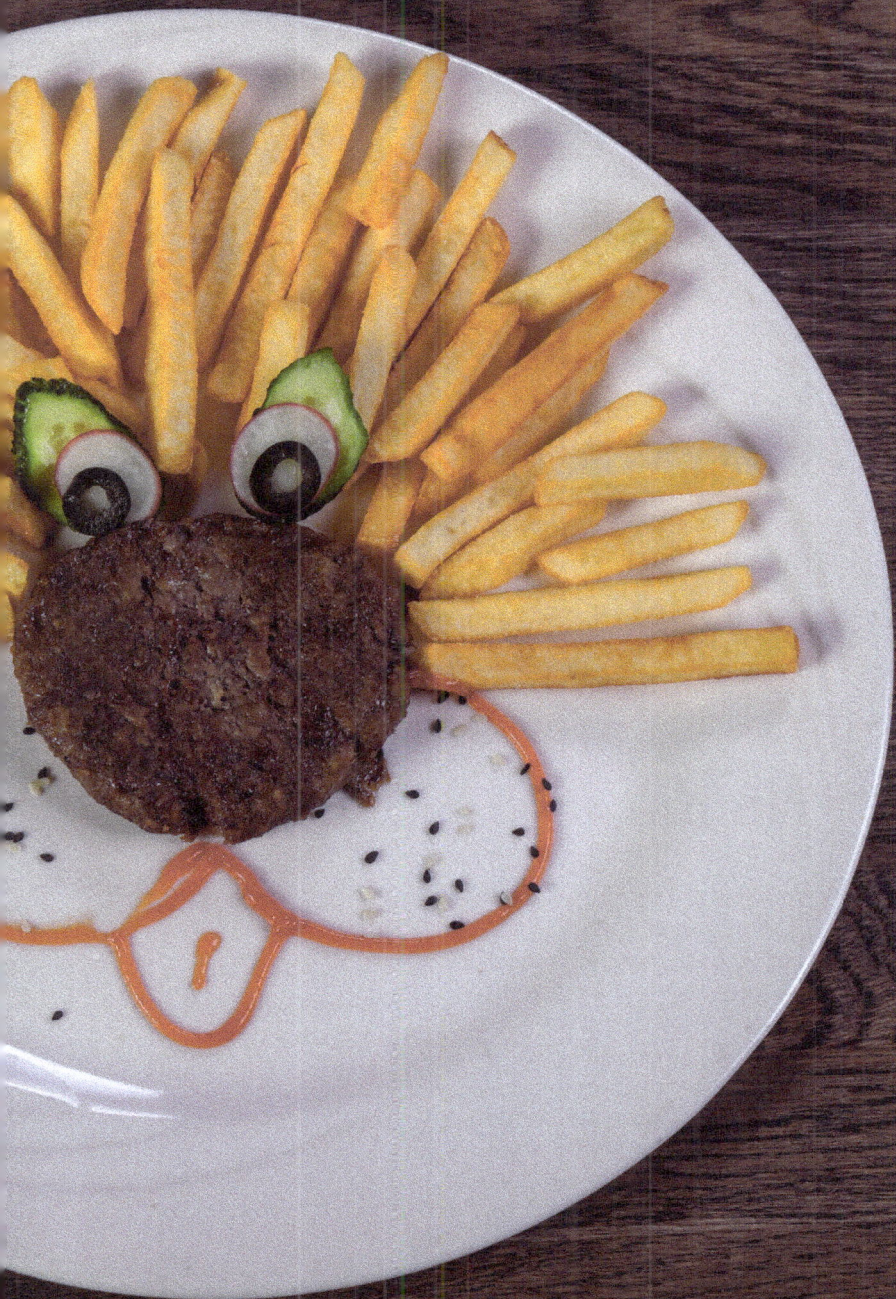

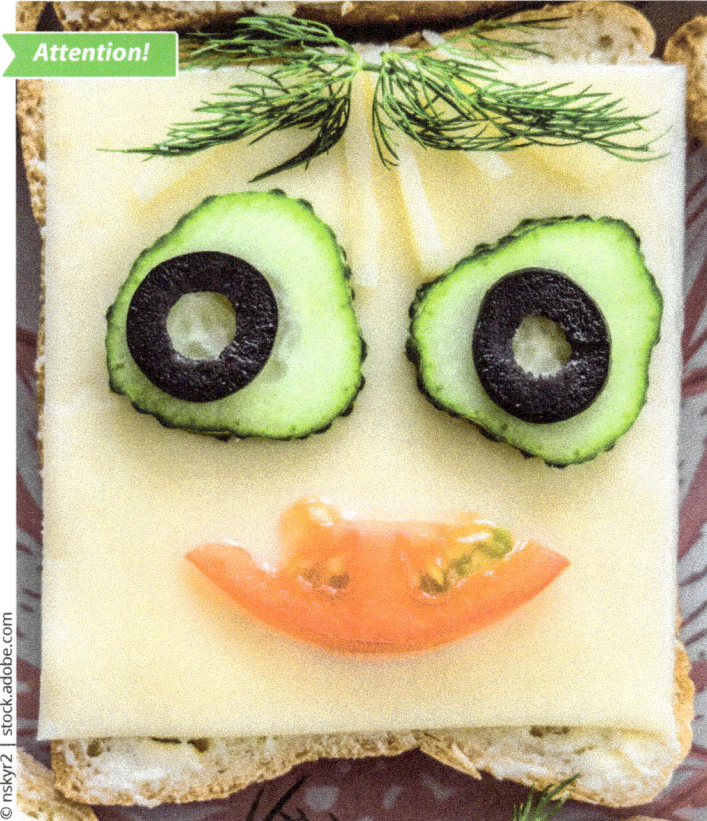

No dill

Inspired by Rena's "Smiley Toast". Its appearance is highly appreciated, especially by children. However, the first thing junior did was throw away the dill. In general, children do not appreciate gourmet decorations with fresh aromatic herbs like dill, parsley, etc. Therefore, we had better leave our crea-tivity for decorating dishes for the grown-ups.

Fresh aromatic herbs are better left out.

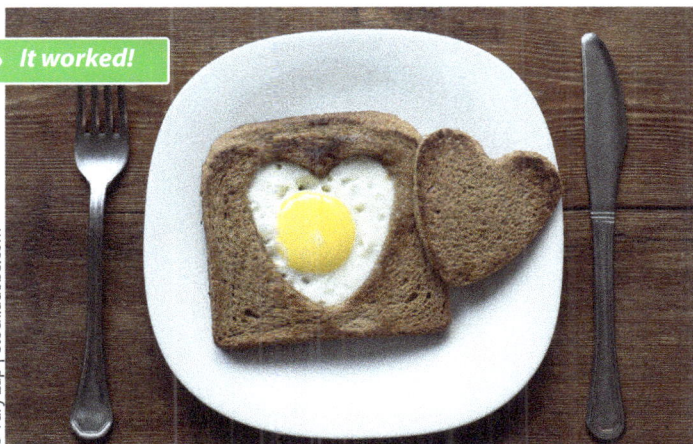

It worked!

© Yury Zap | stock.adobe.com

Simple and safe

We grease a non-stick frying pan lightly and turn the heat on.

We take a bread slice and, using a cookie cutter or a glass, cut a hole in the middle.

We fry one side of the bread lightly and fry the other side a bit more. We flip over the slice in the pan so that the crispier side is up. Next the slice. We also fry both sides of the circle of bread that we cut out.

We fry the egg in the hole in the middle of the bread, as we do with eggs sunny side up. We lower the fire, and cover the pan so that the egg is done properly.

Attention 1: The egg should be as hard as the child likes.

Attention 2: The time for cooking the egg determines how well-done the bottom side of the bread will be.

Idea: You can serve the piece of bread that was cut out with a slice of cheese, tomato, or cucumber.

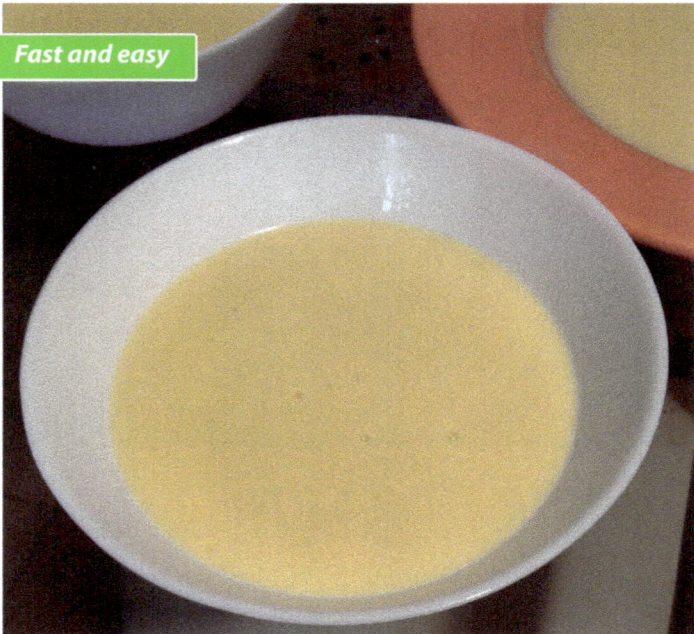

Vanilla custard

We put all the ingredients in a saucepan, without previously warming them up.

We turn the heat on low and vigorously stir so that the corn-flour does not coagulate and the eggs mix nicely. While the mix is still cold, there is no fear of this happening.

When the ingredients are adequately mixed, I turn up the heat and stir vigorously, without stopping until the mixture thickens.

INGREDIENTS

- ½ lit milk
- 2 tsp corn flour
- 1 egg
- ½ cup sugar (or less)
- 1 sachet vanilla
- 1 tsp butter (optional)

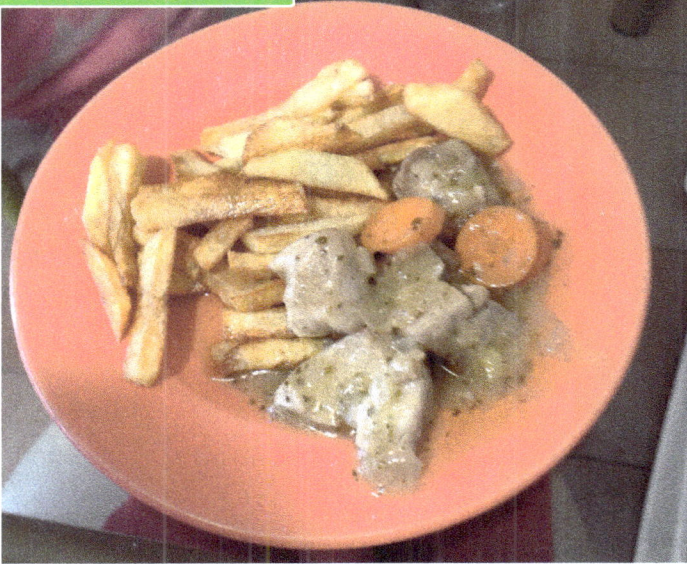

Make them eat carrots

With rice or potatoes

We place all the ingredients, except for the lemon, in a sauce-pan. We add water until the meat is covered. We turn the heat on low and let it simmer until the meat is tender and the sauce thickens.

If we want a thicker sauce, we add 1 tsp of corn flour in the water we added initially to the meat. When the food is cooked, we let it cool, and then we add the lemon and season it.

INGREDIENTS

- ½ kg pork, cut in small cubes
- 1 medium-sized onion
- 1 tsp mustard powder
- 1 tsp oregano
- 3 baby carrots thinly sliced
- 1 lemon, juiced

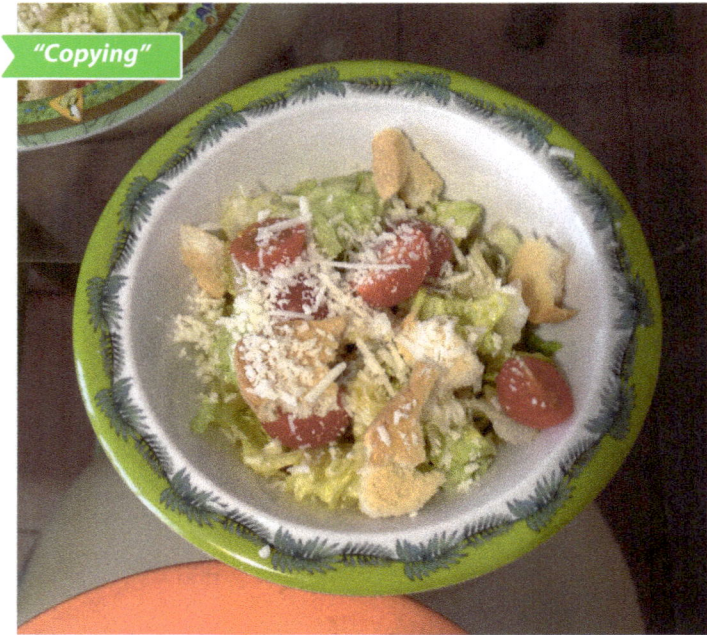

"Copying"

Attractive appearance

It's just a simple salad with lettuce, cherry tomatoes, oil, and lemon.

What makes the difference is the fact that its appearance was adapted to that of a salad that the child ate once at a restaurant and liked.

We merely "copied" the appearance. We added grated cheese and, lacking the croutons and the time, added pieces of toasted bread.

An attractive copy of a Caesar's salad made a humble and straightforward lettuce salad acceptable.

Right "placement"

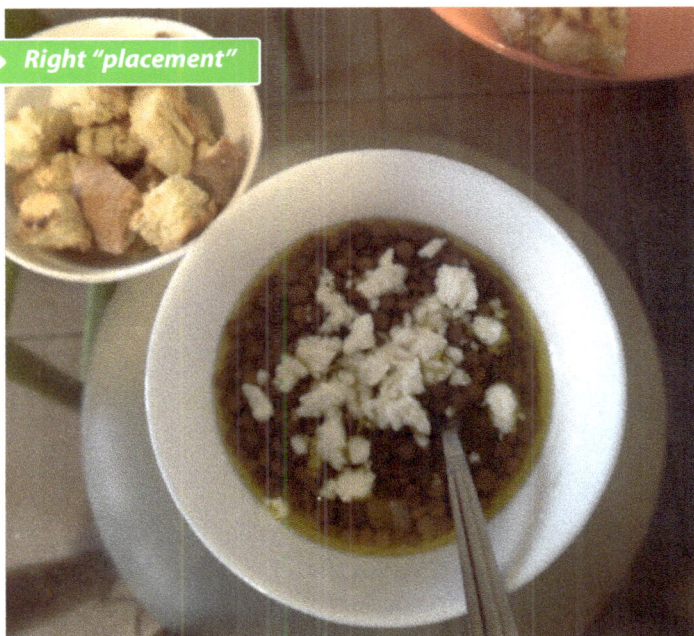

Small quantities

We didn't follow our chef's recipe for lentil mousse.

We put on the table the same lentil soup that we all eat at home but in a smaller quantity and bigger plates and bowls.

We filled the bowl up to the middle then placed it on a bigger shallow dish. The dimensions of the china were disproportionate to the quantity of the food.

We added crumbs of feta because it's the kid's favourite cheese and made croutons out of merely toasted bread.

Eventually, she ate two helpings, which are a regular portion.

....

- What was it that made you eat the lentils today?
- Well, it wasn't but two spoonfuls...
....

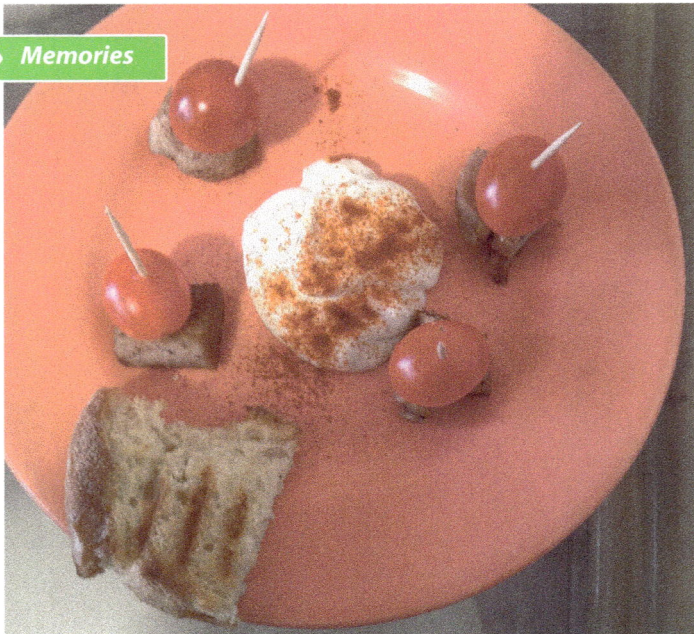

Memories

Brings back great times

Inspired by our chef's "burgers with roast tomatoes", we created a meat dish from yesterday's leftover meat.

We diced it, added half a cherry tomato and stuck them on a toothpick.

In the centre we put a dash of yoghurt sprinkled with paprika for decoration; on the rim, half a toasted slice of bread.

"Dad, this looks like the tidbits we get at the beach! When are you making them again?"

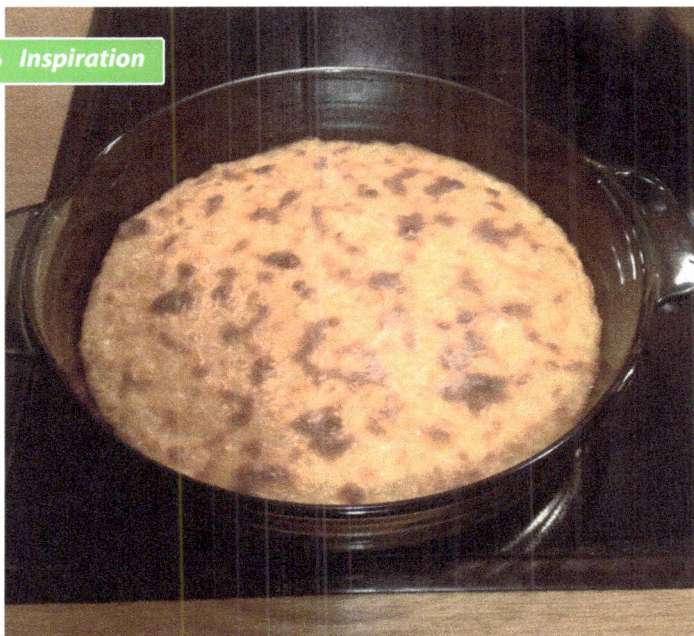

Inspiration

A briam[1] turned into... moussaka[2]

Briam! Not today again! Not with the zucchini and particularly not with these eggplants!

They like moussaka despite the eggplants. So we take the leftover briam, put it in an oven dish and pour béchamel over it. We put it in the oven to cook, and the moussaka is ready!

Béchamel is easy!

In a saucepan we add the ingredients, cold from the fridge: ½ litre of milk, 1 egg, 1 tbsp corn flour and mix vigorously. We turn the heat up and stir until thick. We may add 1 tbsp of butter.

---

1   *See also ratatouille. A vegetable dish consisting usually of onions, courgettes, tomatoes, aubergines, and peppers, fried and stewed (Oxford Dictionary)*

2   *A Greek dish made of minced lamb, aubergines, and tomatoes, with cheese sauce (or Béchamel sauce) on top. (Oxford Dictionary)*

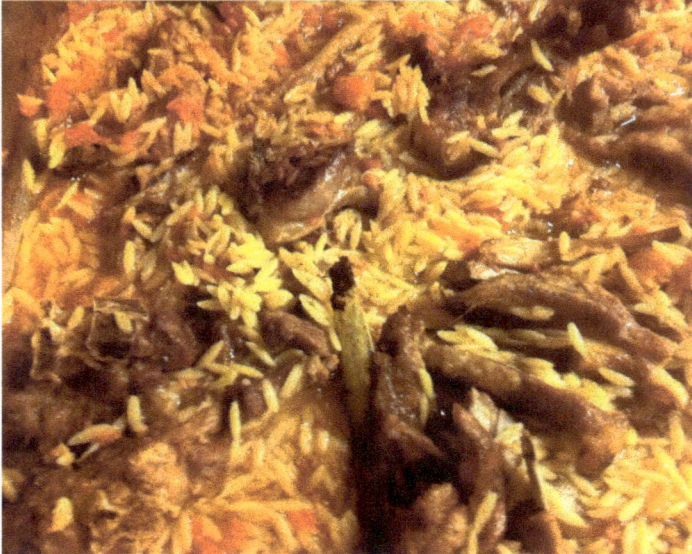

It looks great because I did it myself!

Let's cook together

Like the paediatrician, George Moustakas, points out in his introduction and tips, cooking with the parents can change the whole perspective towards eating from negative into positive.

"Dad, this smells delicious. See the nice colour of the meat!"

This really works. We put our aprons on, we opened our recipe book, and we cooked the pasta together. The children worked along with us throughout the whole procedure, including baking and serving.

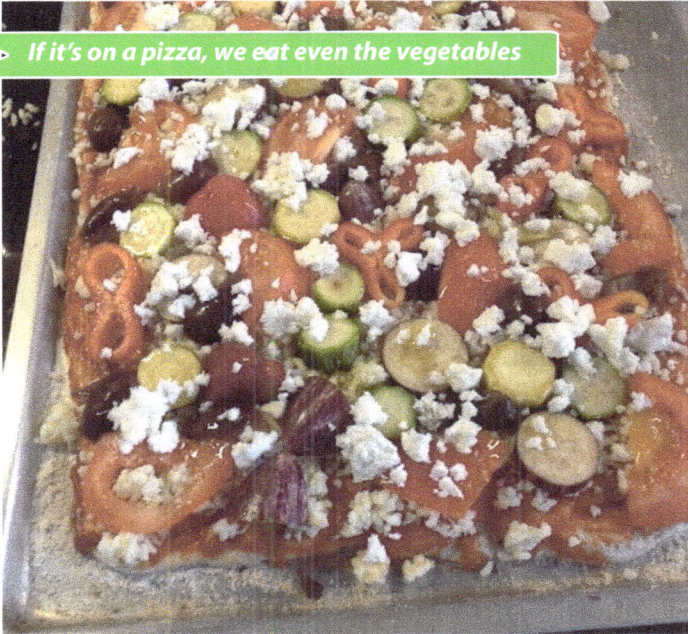

If it's on a pizza, we eat even the vegetables

Pizza with vegetables

This recipe is a variation of our chef's veggie or minced meat pizza. This one consists only of the dough, tomato sauce, and vegetables: tomatoes, zucchini, eggplants and peppers.

We sprinkled it with crushed feta and put it in the oven.

Variation

Instead of tomato sauce, we use minced meat (with tomato) and sprinkled it with grated cheese(s), without the vegetables.

The pieces of tomato are probably in excess since because there is sauce on the crust.

....

Probably the pieces of tomato are in excess since there is sauce on the crust.

....

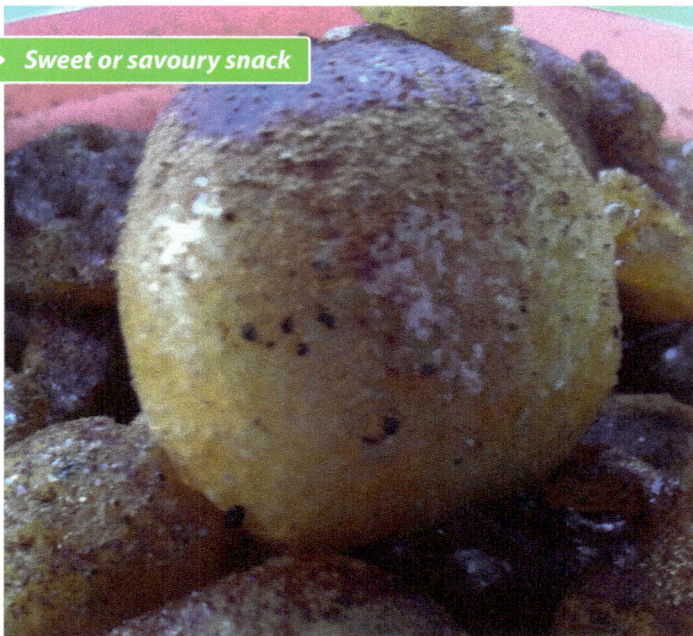

Sweet or savoury snack

Doughnuts

In a bowl, I mix all-purpose flour, cold water and yeast, until the texture becomes a little bit thicker than the batter we use for frying. I cover the bowl with a towel to let it rise. It's better to place it somewhere warm but not too warm; it shouldn't be scorched by the sun. I don't add salt to the mixture.

As soon as the mixture rises and we see blisters, we add the oil to the frying pan or a small saucepan. When the oil is hot, we fill a tablespoon with dough and with our finger we push it into the hot oil. We repeat until the small saucepan is filled with dough balls swimming in oil. As soon as they get a nice blond colour, we remove them from the oil with the help of a slotted spoon.

Serve with feta cheese or as dessert with honey or sugar or cinnamon.

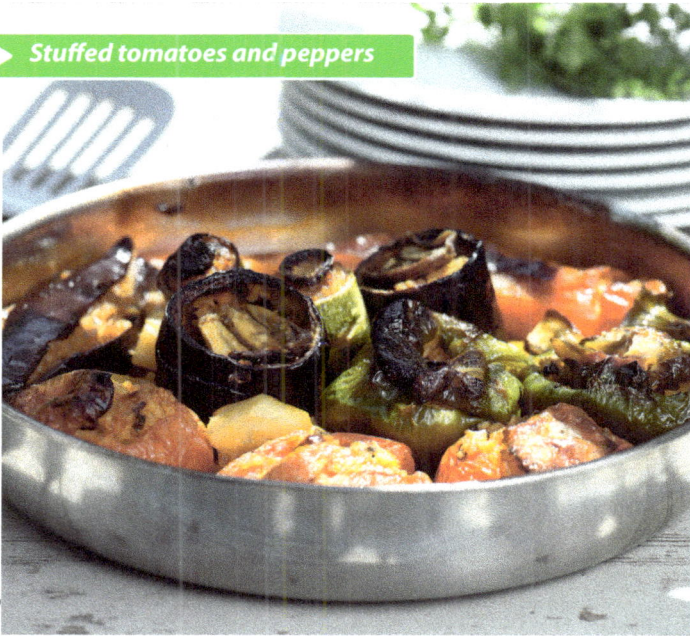

Stuffed tomatoes and peppers

Vangelis Paterakis

The joy of creation

Nothing special. I cut off the tops and show the kids how to empty a tomato and a pepper with the help of a spoon The kids take over the remaining tomatoes and peppers. In a bowl I put two tsp each of sugar, salt and pepper, mint, garlic and finely chopped onion, keeping in mind that 1 tbsp of the mixture will be needed for filling one tomato or pepper. The kids fill the multi with the flesh that was scooped out of the vegetables. When they are ready, I turn the multi on slow to have them cut into pieces. The kids take the bowl of the multi, empty it into the bowl with the rice mixture, and then stir. Now comes the best part! They fill the vegetables with the mix with the help of a tablespoon. Then we pour oil over each vegetable, cover them with their tops, and here is the oven dish, ready for the oven!

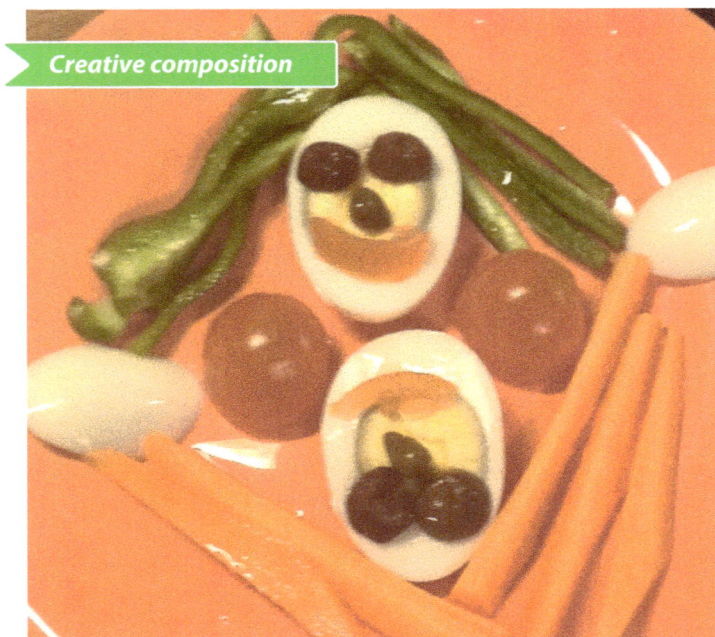

Creative composition

Protein and fibre

It's boiled eggs again, but this time they are slightly different.

Hard-boiled eggers, cut in half, with olives for the eyes, sweet red pepper for the mouth, and strips of carrots and green peppers for the hair.

What is best is the fact that the kids decorated the dish, so I am in no position to tell you what the cherry tomatoes that I can see in the photo on either side of the eggs stand for.

The white things are the whites of another egg.

The food was eaten, and each time the kids created a different figure. I even saw eggs decorated as flying kites!

The great achievement here is the fact that the kids ate the whites of the eggs, while up until now, they would eat only the yolk.

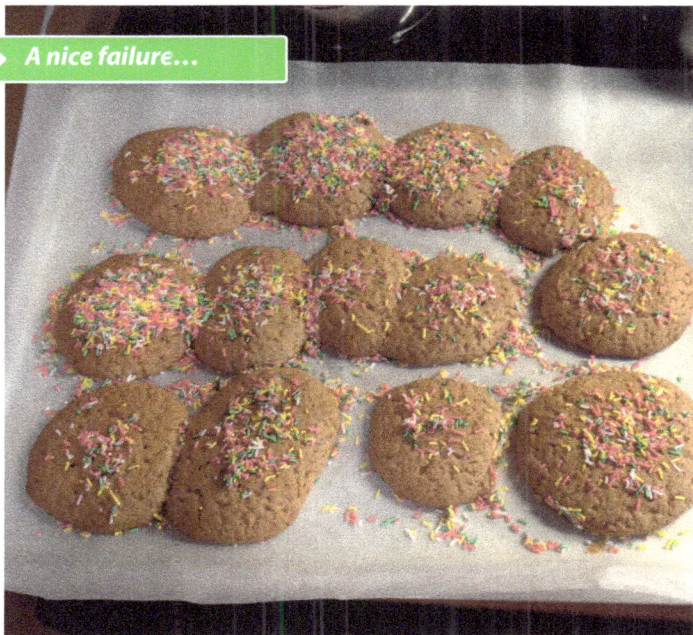

A nice failure…

Interesting experiment

This experiment s confirmation that when the kids participate in cooking and create, miracles happen.

We have here a failed attempt at melomakarona[1]; they were the definition of failure.

We didn't throw them away. We gave the oven dish to the kids and asked them to let their imagination run free. We asked them to improvise. They sprinkled the wannabe melomakarona with multi-coloured toffee and powdered sugar.

The kids were pleased with the result.

It's hard for us, the parents, to understand how they ate them…

---

1 An egg-shaped Greek dessert made mainly from flour, olive oil, and honey (Anon, 2018)

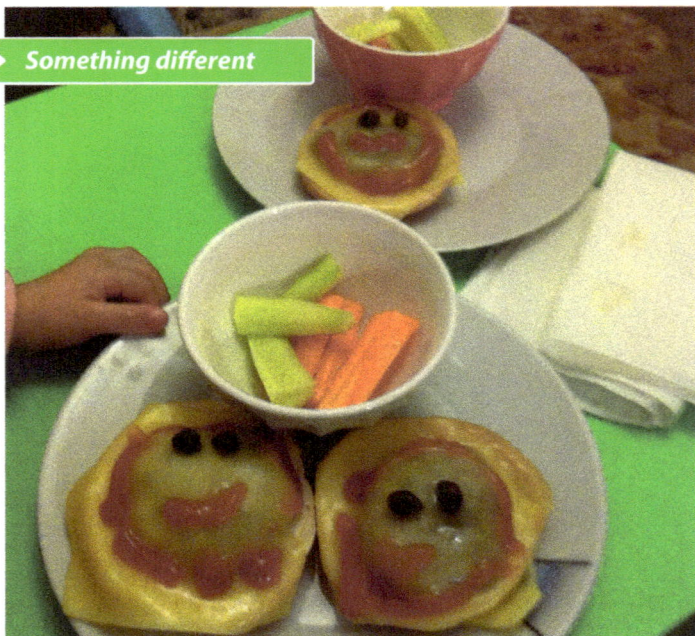

Something different

Smiley pizzas

You read about the pizza with minced meat, and you remember all about it.

Instead of dough, we used bread; instead of minced meat, leftover burgers. We heated them in the oven for a while (the dish was placed on the bottom of the oven so that the bread could roast).

While still hot from the oven, we added sliced cheese, which melted. We added olives for the eyes and homemade ketchup for the mouth and decoration.

I cut carrots and cucumber in strips, put them in a bowl, and add vinegar.

We put them on a tray that we took to the living room where we watched our favourite movie, munching away on this snack.

A different breakfast

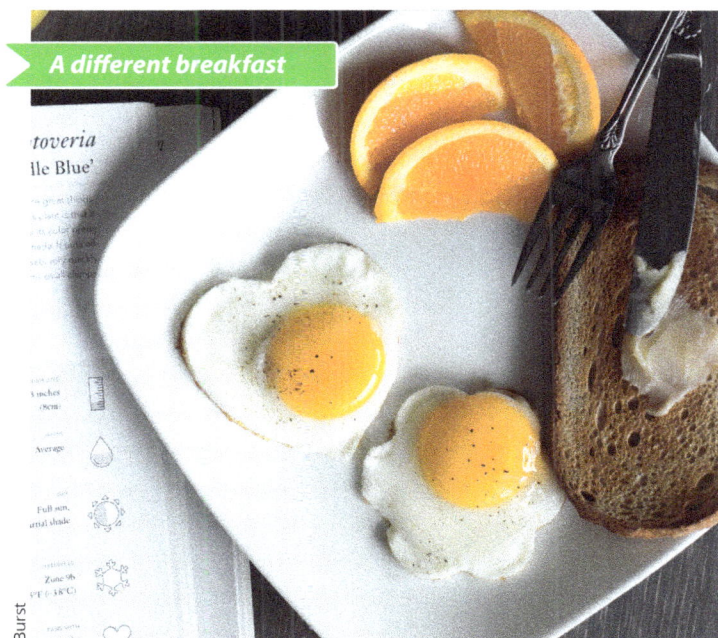

Eggs and fruit

These cookie cutters for the Christmas biscuits work miracles; they help achieve a nice shape for fried eggs, sunny side up.

This time, there was another contributing factor: we ate this breakfast on one of our trips abroad. We concluded

that what the parents say does not count much; it's seeing their friends eat it that matters more.

This is why we decided to offer a similar breakfast, but we made it even better. Not only did we add orange slices, bread, and butter, we also gave shape to the eggs.

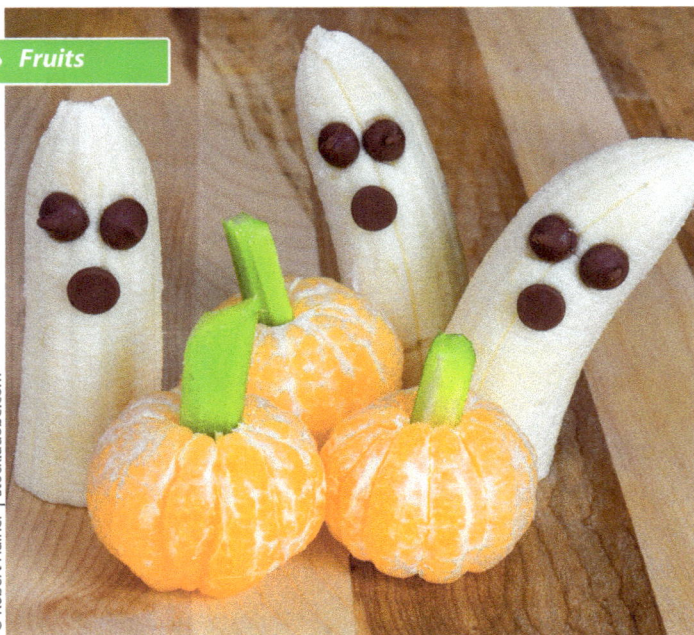

Fruits

© Robert Hainer | stock.adobe.com

Ideas from Halloween

Bananas and chocolate spread, apples with cinnamon and honey, orange with cinnamon...

Kids get bored quickly; this is why imagination is of the essence.

What would you say to banana "ghosts" and orange or tangerine "pumpkins"?

Thankfully, there was a Halloween party that inspired us to "dress up" our fruit in the Halloween spirit.

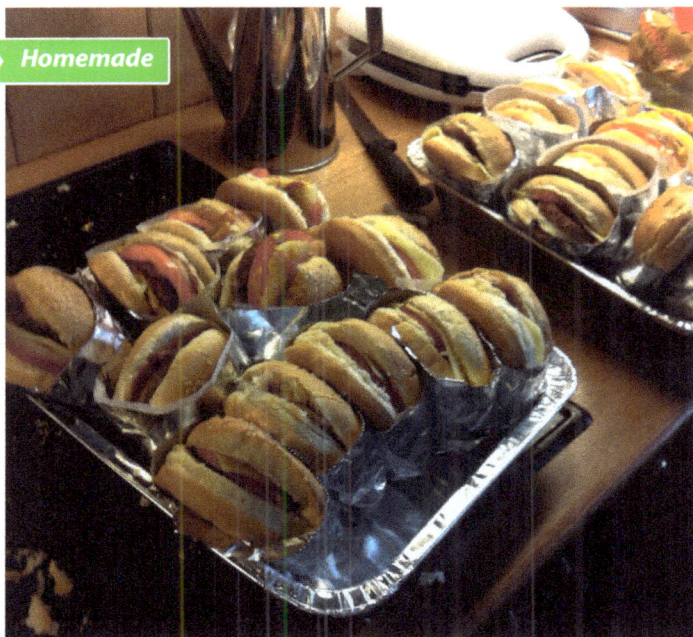

Homemade

Hamburgers for parties

Now that I grew up, I agree that you cannot have a party without soda drinks and chips.

However, we may add something that the kids love:

Mini hamburgers! We take small buns, cut them in half, fill each with home-made ketchup, a slice of cheese, a homemade (thin) hamburger, a tomato slice, and here they are!

We wrap them in kitchen paper and foil, to help kids handle the ingredients of the filling without making a mess.

Very easy

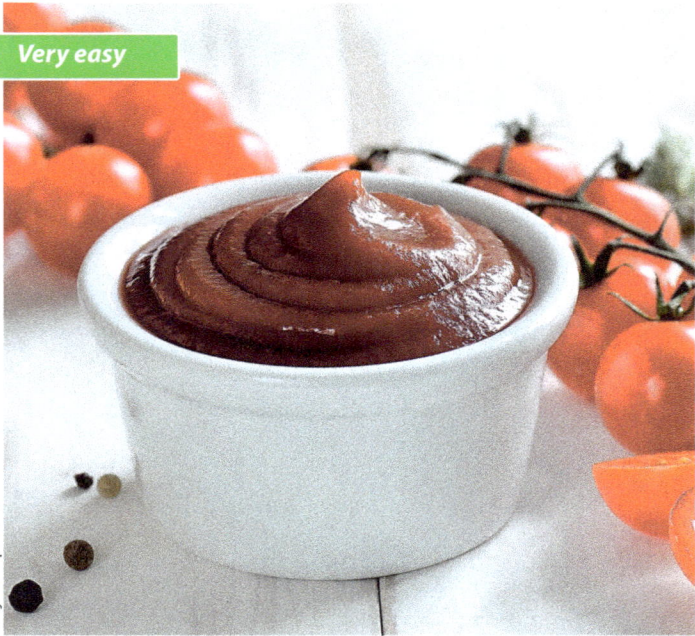

fortyforks | stock.adobe.com

Homemade ketchup

It's the same as making a sauce, but without the garlic and onion.

In a saucepan you put half a cup of oil, half a cup of vinegar, 2 tbsp sugar and 1 tin of tomato juice (approx. 300 g).

You bring to a simmer, and you often stir until all the liquid is gone and you have a smooth, thick sauce. You try it for salt, pepper, or vinegar. You can add more tomato juice to cover up too much vinegar.

Let the sauce cool, put in a jar and store in the fridge.

This sauce lasts for a long time in the fridge as salt, sugar, and vinegar are natural preservatives.

Interesting to read

Meal ideas

By NHS Choices (Appendix 4, *page 135*)

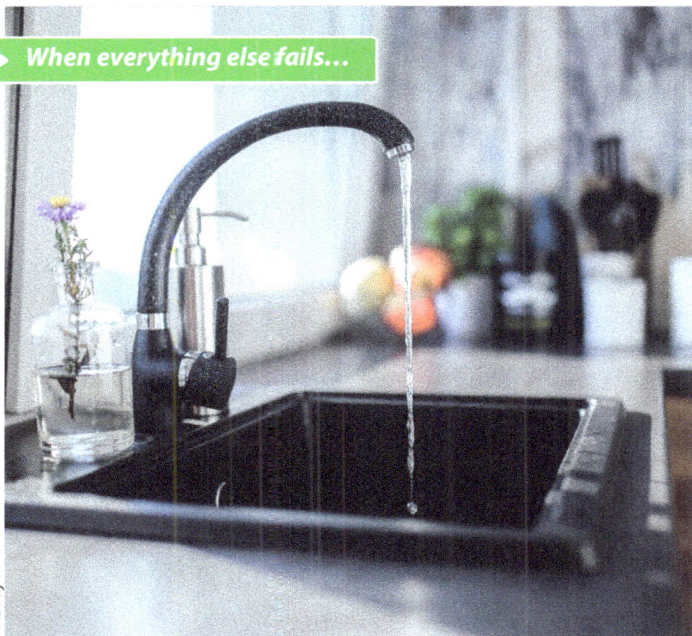

When everything else fails...

Pixabay

Let's go to the sink

Particularly around the age of 2, when all of our tricks have failed and we find ourselves at our wit's end, we go for the big trick.

We place the child on a stool suitable for their age, as close to the rim of the sink as possible.

Give them an apron (or a pinafore) to put on. Fill the sink with plastic dishes, spoons, and forks and ask them to help us with the washing up.

The idea is to keep the child busy, to make it relax, but to avoid at all costs giving the impression that we are at play. On the contrary, we are doing serious work here, and the child gets its fair share of the job at hand. And, as the water runs and the suds get foamy, the child concentrates on the job, and the parent tricks it into eating. I don't know if this works for everybody, but with us it was a big hit.

Section 4

A true story.

The torture of eating and the psychiatrist's comment.

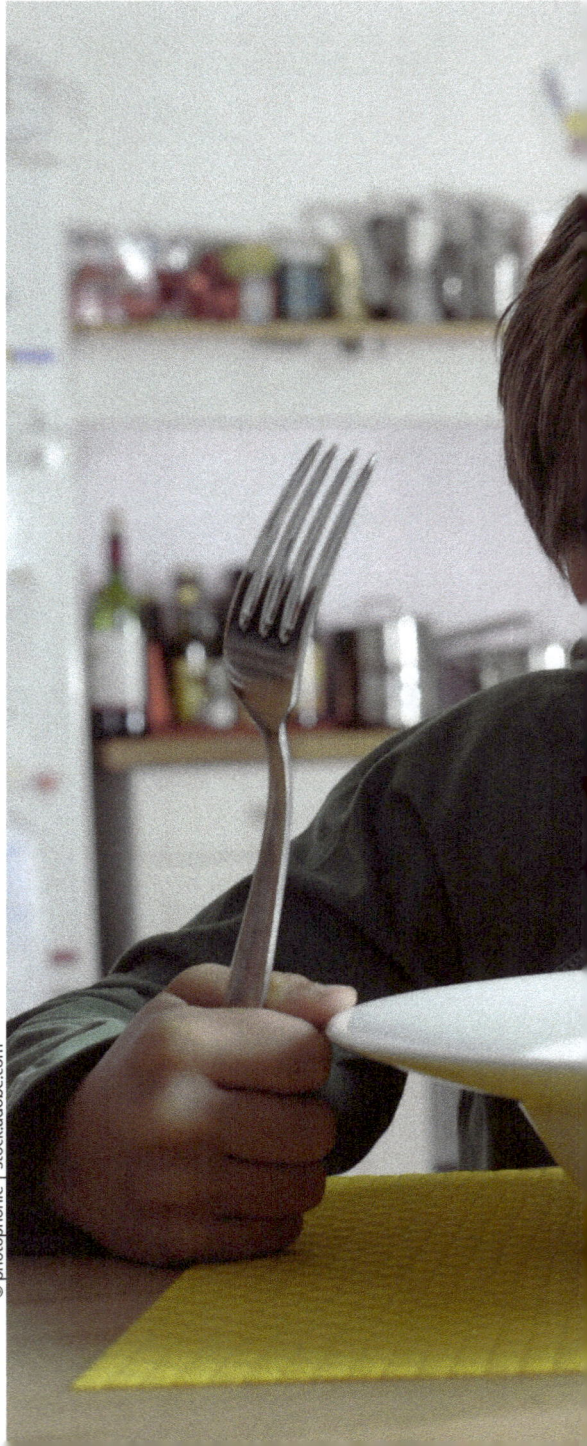

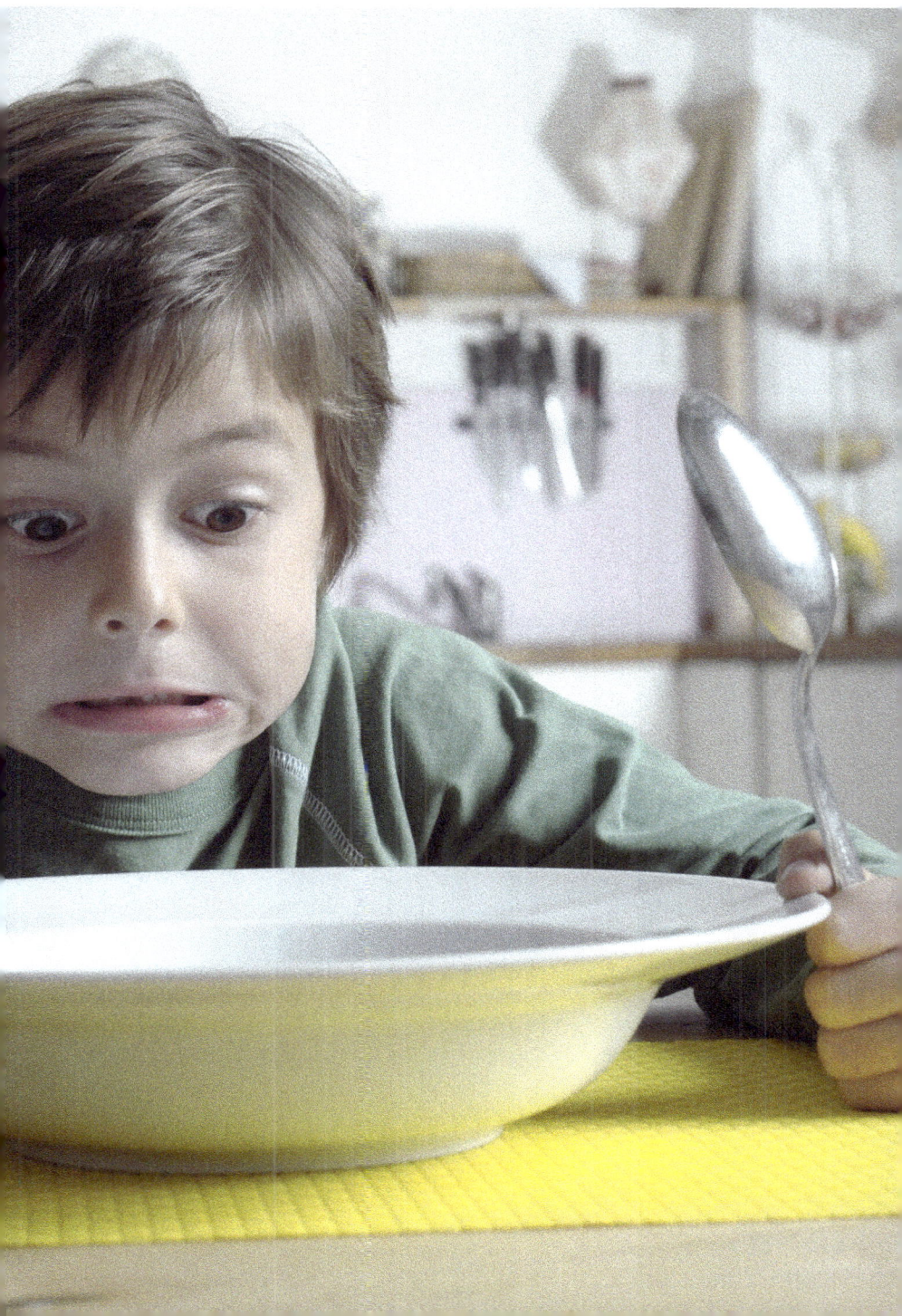

Putting an end to the torture of eating after 35 years

A father analyses his own experience with an eating disorder as a child

LEONIDAS STERGIOU

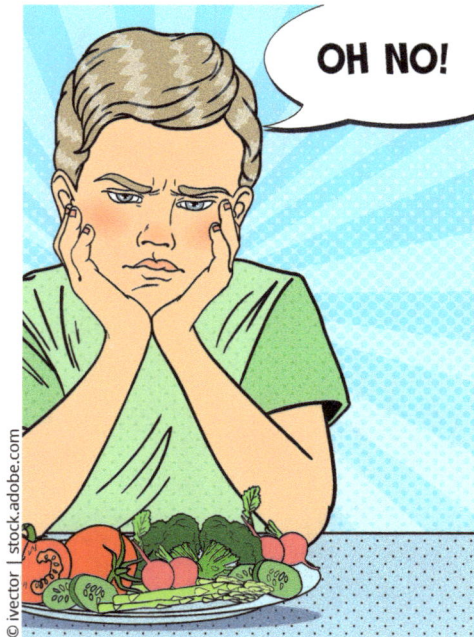

© ivector | stock.adobe.com

From childhood until I finished elementary school, I remember that there was this knot in the pit of my stomach: the disgust I felt for almost all kinds of food, and the real torture I went through whenever it was mealtime at home. Adolescence came along, and things changed; I went to another school where I made new friends. The need to socialise—to become part of a new team—and the need to earn the approval of my peers were factors that might have contributed to the solution to the problem. Maybe my parents' efforts paid off, or perhaps it was my internal need to overcome my misery. Perhaps the key was just adolescence. Or maybe a little bit of all of these.

I had been taken to all kinds of doctors, looking for pathological, physical or psychological problems.

Up until that time, I was what my granddad used to call "one of these children who can go without food forever, never getting hungry, feeding on empty air..."

I will try to describe myself as a child from the first day that I can remember. I need to share with you the feelings of a healthy child who does not want to eat and thus becomes fussy about food. Mainly, however, I want the experts to use my experience to decode the psychological background of the problem in order to find the mistakes and offer advice to parents – the readers.

Guilt

Eating time was a torturous time, not only for me but for the entire family and mostly for my mother. I still remember her desperate efforts. Appetizers, treats, French fries, sweets, all in vain! At best I would eat something I liked and then I would throw it up; it came automatically, not necessarily accompanied by feelings of revulsion. I still remember my mother's frustration, but also her love at times like this.

I had been taken to all kinds of doctors, looking for pathological, physical, or psychological problems. All those visits, all those tests, all in vain, all negative; nothing was ever found. I was entirely healthy; the blood tests came up a marvel. My grandfather, who was also my paediatrician, told my mother: "Don't worry; there is nothing wrong with the child. Let him eat only the things he fancies, and little by little his appetite will catch up with him; he will find his way. And there will come a time when he will pray to lose his appetite so that the girls will be attracted to his body".

"Let him eat only the things he fancies, and little by little his appetite will catch up with him; he will find his way."

A difficult equation

It sounded nice, but there was an almost insurmountable obstacle: There was almost nothing I liked. Neither the French fries nor the souvlaki appealed to me! The grease on the pita was so disgusting! The smell and the fat on the meat made me want to puke.

What I eat

What did I eat with pleasure? I eat mainly dairy products, such as milk, yoghurt, and cheeses. Second best was the egg (only hard-boiled, with salt and pepper, never fried, because I had this idea that the white would show, uncooked – it reminded me of mucus). Then, there was bread, which I liked to eat with feta cheese, oil, and oregano or with butter and sugar, but that was rare and always on the sly, as sugar and butter were not considered healthy foods for children. I also liked spaghetti without meat – at most, with tomato sauce and grated cheese. For dessert, I prefer custard, ice cream, and white-cream cakes – no chocolate whatsoever.

This was the list of foods that my mother had to work. I didn't eat fruits, vegetables, meat, or fish. The only exceptions to the rule were Grandma Eleni's burger and my mother's meatballs. The burger was tasty, succulent, and redolent of the aromas of lemon and oregano, never reeking of meat. I used to wrap it in a pita with yoghurt. The meatball was crunchy, soft, smelling of garlic and mint, never small or dry.

I was mainly eating dairy products such as milk, yoghurt, and cheeses.

I was not that particular when eating out, at an aunt's for instance or at a tavern. This brought about comments from my family, or rather complaints, that "I preferred the food prepared by strangers to homemade food" and, similar to that, that "I preferred the junk food of the taverns and restaurants to homemade food". I found this annoying, so I made up my mind, I would be difficult when eating out as well. Besides, I don't remember ever being hungry.

The comparison and the... veal's head

But what I found most annoying were my father's comments, who was a lover of traditional foods such as tripe, trotters, boiled goat and veal's head soup. Out of love for me but to what a cost, he loved to compare his healthy traditional eating habits to ours, us being the "sterilised" city kids who would not order veal's head but spaghetti without sauce or burgers at the taverns. I was in turmoil; particularly when I had to watch my younger brother eat with relish almost everything, chewing the meat of the cheeks of the veal's head while I threw up.

However, my grandfather the paediatrician's advice and my mother's perseverance and character (she is a fighter for the freedom and the respect of the personality of the others) were sufficient. It took time, but in the end, they worked.

The beginning of the end to the problem

My mother's stress over my eating subsided; she stopped nagging me to make sure that I ate. She imposed the same attitude on my grandmother, and, with hindsight I can say now, to all the family, my dad included: "Let him eat whatever he wants," which was the ultimatum.

After having assuaged my hunger for my favourite foods, and while the others were eating what they usually did, gradually I started inserting more foods into my diet.

Miracles do not happen overnight but for this universal change in attitude: "we support Leonida's special preferences," paid in the long run.

After having assuaged my hunger for my favourite foods and while the others were eating what they usually did, I gradually started inserting more foods into my diet. I started with chicken, either in the oven with potatoes or on the spit. Then came steaks, without the fat of course. The rest of the meats followed, with the fat removed with a surgeon's precision. Then followed the foods in tomato sauce, briam, the eggplants, the green peas in tomato sauce, and lentils. Later the remaining foods followed, except the okra and of course the tripe, the veal's head, and the trotters. These and the fat remain excluded from my diet up to now.

The process was not easy. Many a time I went through phases of false attractions and quite often I had to go back to my previous preferences before the list of the foods I liked became clear. For example, I wanted to try artichokes only to find that I didn't like them. I went back to my initial choices until one day I tried artichokes again and I loved them. My menu gets enriched with new foods, little by little.

The process was not easy. Many a time I went through phases of false attractions, and quite often I had to go back to my previous preferences before the list of the foods I liked became clear.

Today I feel comfortable about eating. I know what I don't eat, and I avoid it. I also know the foods that I can eat, as the case might be, although I am not a great fan of them. For example, I can live without sausages. I know which foods I prefer to others; for instance, I prefer vegetables and fish to meat. At the same time I am well aware of the fact that I must maintain a balanced diet, so I eat meat too, but only when it's cooked to my liking; if it's not, I make do with my salad, and leave the meat for another time. I am still selective about eating. I don't eat for eating's sake; I want to enjoy my food. If this cannot happen—if I cannot enjoy my plate due to bad cooking, lack of time, or lousy-quality ingredients—I choose to eat the minimum possible that will keep me going, for example, bread and cheese, yoghurt, milk, etc.

"Self-analysis"

While writing my story with the aim of helping and inspiring parents to understand their fussy kids better, I went through a stage of "self-analysis".

The first step was to recall from memory: to describe and analyse my own experience meticulously. I put pen to paper and started writing down feelings, symptoms, possible causes, and effective and ineffective techniques.

The second step was to draw a sort of map of the "problem" in an attempt to distinguish the problem from the symptom.

The best days of my life were the ones when, for whatever reason, food was delayed, or we resorted to snacks.

I created three categories (circles) of possible causes and solutions. This classification was not based on scientific data or statistics but solely on my understanding.

Stress

The first category included psychological factors, so I named it "Stress". I tried to analyse the possible reasons for the unrelenting knot at the pit of my stomach.

Behaviour

The second category was called "Behaviour" and included all the inherent characteristics of an individual's personality and the (unique) way they react to the environment and new experiences. Here I analysed my indifference towards food and why the best days of my life were the ones when, for whatever reason, food was delayed or we resorted to snacks.

Cooking

I gave the title "Cooking" to the section where I listed all my preferences regarding taste and presentation of each dish. For instance, I like spaghetti

I have my own preferences; therefore, why shouldn't children have their own?

Bolognese; however, I want the sauce thick, with a velvety texture, juicy and spicy. I am loath to add cheese to such a nice minced-meat sauce because it blurs its taste and cheese also makes it saltier.

Conclusion, I have my own preferences; therefore, why shouldn't children have their own?

The psychiatrist's comment

Reading my friend Lecnida's story, I couldn't help conjuring up in my mind the picture of the kid sitting at the table while his father consumes the veal's head. On the one hand, little Leonidas wants to be like his father but cannot cope with the veal's head. However, he perceives his new-born brother as a threat since the entire family is focused on the newcomer and his needs.

Crafty Leonidas is left with no other choice but to refuse food. Either way, his mother would never let him go hungry. Using extreme selectiveness in food as his tool, little Leonidas becomes once again the focal point of the family. There is nothing but doctors, tests, and exclusive cooking for fussy little Leonidas while the little brother plays at being the good kid and eats the veal's head.

Rivalries and struggles for love and attention in the closed circuit that is family.

Pavlos Sakkas, *professor of psychiatry, National and Kapodistrian University of Athens*

Section 5

Guide.

Expert tips.

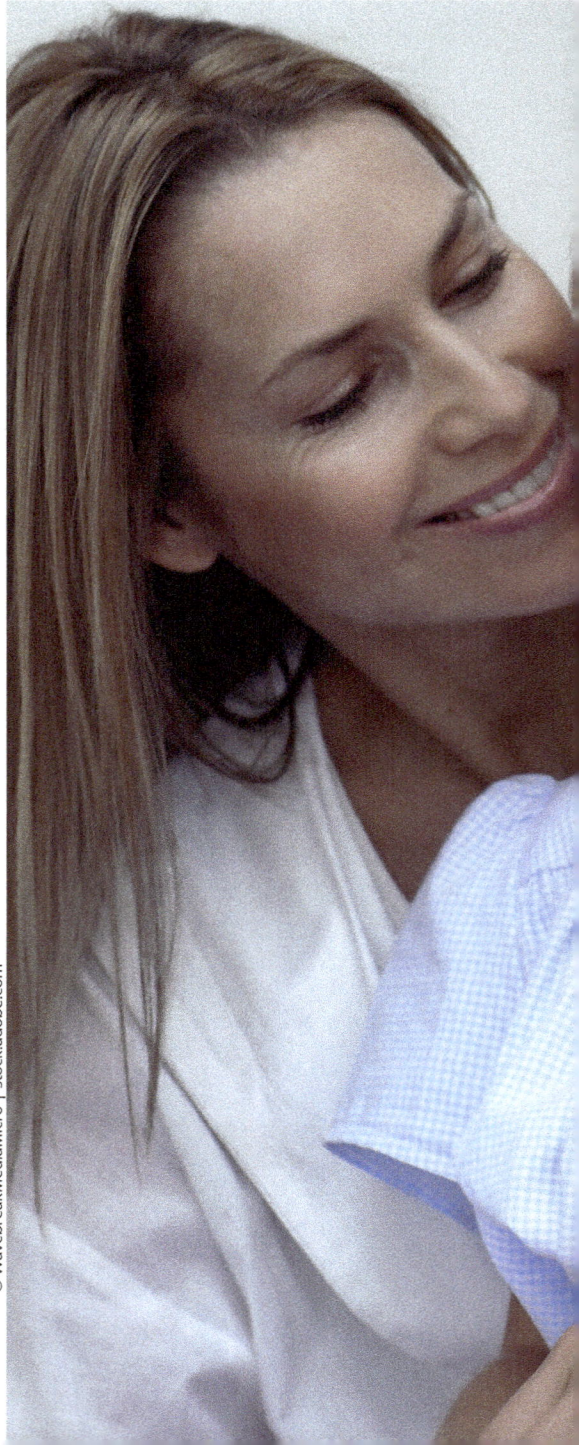

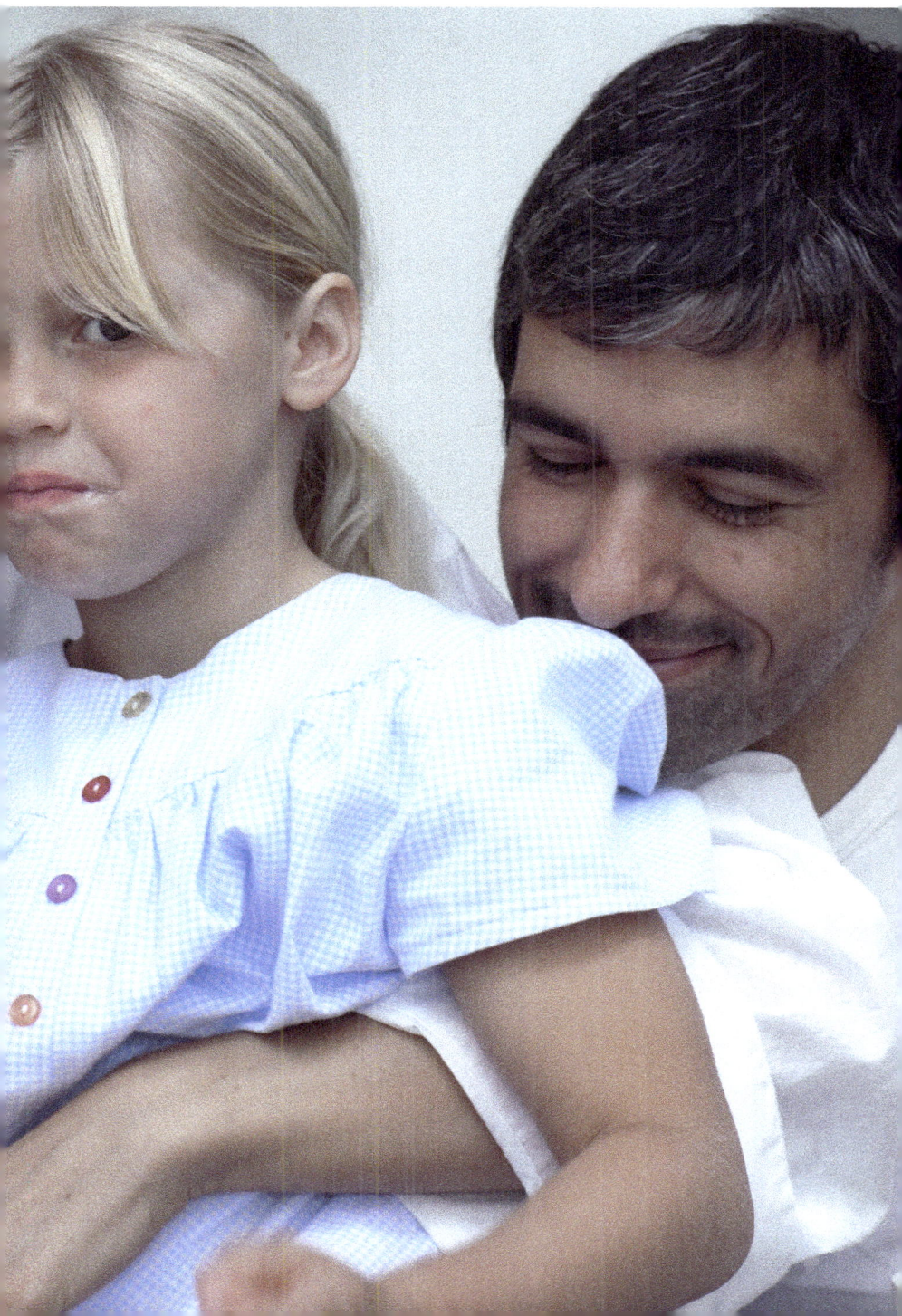

Fifteen useful tips

*And much more that you must discover
with the help of the experts*

1 **No stress, no hysterics, and no panic.** No guilt. Not everything is the parent's fault, nor can he or she solve all problems, and nor is he or she God. The parent is not to be placed under continuous evaluation. Relaxed, smiling parents put children at ease, infusing them with confidence, not insecurity.

2 **We offer tasty foods,** always keeping in mind the child's preferences. Do you eat everything, regardless of the way they are cooked?

3 **A beautiful presentation matters a lot.** We have to be resourceful. Colours, shapes, and small quantities for the size of the plate help considerably. Instead of serving two spoonfuls in a small dish, try putting them in a big plate, and add a dash of colour (e.g., carrot, pepper); you will see, it makes a world of difference.

4 **The children eat and drink with their parents,** even if it happens only once a day or, at least, some days of the week.

5 **Parents and their offspring,** except for babies, eat and drink the same stuff. Instead of wine, the children may

dr nk juice that matches the colour of their parents' beverage.

6 **The parents should enjoy their food and make it obvious.** If, when eating, you grumble about something, if you quarrel with the wife and the in-laws, or if you are on the phone, why would you expect the child to like it?

7 **Routine, schedule and discipline.** Eating at all times, being fed by different people, at different houses, increase the children's feeling of stress and insecurity. The children should eat at the same place, at the same house, at the same hours and with the same people. Routine helps kids control anxiety.

8 **We don't associate eating with fear**, punishment, reward (presents, toys, rides, etc.), and games during the meals.

9 **We motivate the child** but subtly, so that the child does not perceive motivation as a reward for eating. The only reward should be the pleasure of enjoying a good meal.

10 **We stimulate the appetite and the reward mechanism** allowing them from time to time to eat something they crave for even if it is not considered quite healthy (e.g., a slice of pizza or cake or, in any case, something they are fond of). **All in moderation**, all in balance, all with consistency. Some "bad" foods or ingredients may not be considered healthy. However, they are not poisonous. As stated above, all in moderation, under the guidance of the experts. With their help, we draft a "cost and benefit" spreadsheet for our choices. Each decision and each technique must aim at a strategy. We make sure that the positive results outnumber the negative ones. Among the positive ones, we include the child's mental balance, the pleasure, the relaxation, the training, and the creation of sweet memories with the parents. Sometimes, we have to counterbalance the good with the bad ones—bad ones being, for instance, sugar, cold meats, or a little bit more salt.

11 **I teach my child to learn**, to set boundaries, to experiment, to tell the difference between right and wrong, wrong and dangerous, bad and worst. And also to protect him or herself from danger. The messages must be simple and clear according to the child's age and character. You can say that a lesson makes sense when the recipient perceives and decodes it correctly. Interference from the environment is not allowed.

12 **I learn, and I spend time with my child**. Try to walk in their shoes; recall how you were as a child: how you perceived the world when you were their age.

13 **Life is good.** We enjoy life; we eat together, drink together, watch TV together, and go on holidays all together. We are sad together, and then we laugh again together. We are a team, and we love and support each other. Let's make the best of it. And if today brings something terrible or sad, tomorrow will bring something good. Provided we are ready to recognise it for what it is and grab it.

14 **Educating the parent:** It takes reading and discussions with the experts.

15 **Love**, caring, communication, warmth, security, creativity, and tons of hugs!

There are preferences

"The three most frequently refused food groups were shellfish, beans, and vegetables, and the three least refused food groups were fish, fruits, and eggs. Children required foods to be prepared in a certain way—mainly for shellfish and beans. Only 3% of children required eggs to be prepared in a certain way. Fish was not likely to be refused; however, it was required to be prepared in a certain way.

if children could find an appropriate preparation for disliked foods then they might choose to eat the foods with the preparation. These findings imply that an appropriate food preparation method that positively influences food intake would be helpful for the prevention of poor growth"

(Kwon et al., 2017)

Fig. 4. The proportion % of children who usually refused a specific food group

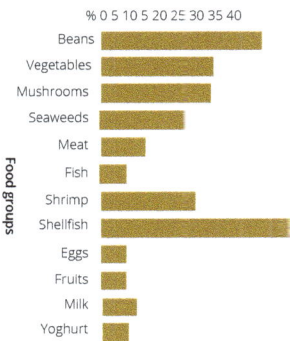

Fig. 5. The proportion % of children who usually requested food preparation in a certain way for each food group

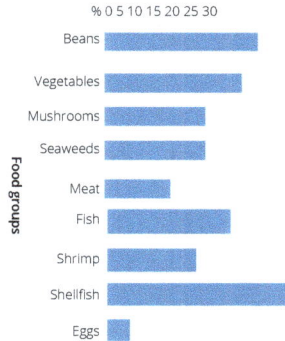

Fig 4 and fig. 5: Kwon, K., Shim, J., Kang, M. and Paik, H.-Y. (2017)

123

Glossary

Anorexia nervosa: An emotional disorder characterised by an obsessive desire to lose weight by refusing to eat.

Eating disorder: Any of a range of psychological disorders characterised by abnormal or disturbed eating habits (e.g., anorexia nervosa).

Fussy eating: Usually, a toddler's sudden refusal to eat many different foods. Fussy eating is a phase that most toddlers go through, often in their second year of life.

Neophobic behaviour: Fear of new foods and food rejection related to a limited preference for all food groups. Neophobic behaviour is especially common regarding vegetables and fruits.

Picky eaters: For the purposes of this book, children who refuse more than two food groups.

Picky eating behaviour: Includes eating a small amount of food, eating a limited variety of foods, displaying neophobic behaviour, refusing to eat specific food groups, and preferring a particular food preparation method.

Sources:
BabyCentre UK (2015), Kwon et. al, (2016). *See also references.*

Appendix 1

Dealing with child behaviour problems

There are lots of possible reasons for difficult behaviour in toddlers and young children.

Often it's just because they're tired, hungry, overexcited, frustrated or bored.

How to handle difficult behaviour

If problem behaviour is causing you or your child distress, or upsetting the rest of the family, it's important to deal with it.

Do what feels right

What you do has to be right for your child, yourself and the family. If you do something you don't believe in or that you don't feel is right, it probably won't work. Children notice when you don't mean what you're saying.

Don't give up

Once you've decided to do something, continue to do it. Solutions take time to work. Get support from your partner, a friend, another parent or your health visitor. It's good to have someone to talk to about what you're doing.

Be consistent

Children need consistency. If you react to your child's behaviour in one way one day and a different way the next, it's confusing for them. It's also important that everyone close to your child deals with their behaviour in the same way.

Try not to overreact

This can be difficult. When your child does something annoying time after time, your anger and frustration can build up.

It's impossible not to show your irritation sometimes, but try to stay calm. Move on to other things you can both enjoy or feel good about as soon as possible.

Find other ways to cope with your frustration, like talking to other parents.

Talk to your child

Children don't have to be able to talk to understand. It can help if they understand why you want them to do something. For example, explain why you want them to hold your hand while crossing the road.

Once your child can talk, encourage them to explain why they're angry or upset. This will help them feel less frustrated.

Be positive about the good things

When a child's behaviour is difficult, the things they do well can be overlooked. Tell your child when you're pleased about something they've done. You can let your child know when you're pleased by giving them attention, a hug or a smile.

Offer rewards

You can help your child by rewarding them for behaving well. For example, praise them or give them their favourite food for tea.

If your child behaves well, tell them how pleased you are. Be specific. Say something like, "Well done for putting your toys back in the box when I asked you to."

Don't give your child a reward before they've done what they were asked to do. That's a bribe, not a reward.

Avoid smacking

Smacking may stop a child doing what they're doing at that moment, but it doesn't have a lasting positive effect.

Children learn by example so, if you hit your child, you're telling them that hitting is okay. Children who are treated aggressively by their parents are more likely to be aggressive themselves. It's better to set a good example instead.

Things that can affect your child's behaviour

Life changes – any change in a child's life can be difficult for them. This could be the birth of a new baby, moving house, a change of childminder, starting playgroup or something much smaller.

You're having a difficult time – children are quick to notice if you're feeling upset or there are problems in the family. They may behave badly when you feel least able to cope. If you're having problems don't blame yourself, but don't blame your child either if they react with difficult behaviour.

How you've handled difficult behaviour before – sometimes your child may react in a particular way because of how you've handled a problem in the past. For example, if you've given your child sweets to keep them quiet at the shops, they may expect sweets every time you go there.

Needing attention – your child might see a tantrum as a way of getting attention, even if it's bad attention. They may wake up at night because they want a cuddle or some company. Try to give them more attention when they're behaving well and less when they're being difficult.

NHS Choices
www.nhs.uk

Used by permission.

Appendix 2

Fussy eaters

It's natural to worry whether your child is getting enough food if they refuse to eat sometimes.

But it's perfectly normal for toddlers to refuse to eat or even taste new foods.

The trick is not to worry about what your child eats in a day or if they don't eat everything at mealtimes. It's more helpful to think about what they eat over a week.

If your child is active and gaining weight, and they seem well, then they're getting enough to eat.

As long as your child eats some food from the 4 main food groups (fruit and vegetables; potatoes, bread, rice, pasta and other starchy carbohydrates; dairy or dairy alternatives; and beans, pulses, fish, eggs, meat and other proteins) you don't need to worry.

Gradually introduce other foods and keep going back to the foods your child didn't like before. Children's tastes change. One day they'll hate something, but a month later they may love it.

Keep offering a variety of foods – it may take lots of attempts before your child accepts some foods.

Tips for parents of fussy eaters

- Give your child the same food as the rest of the family, but remember not to add salt to your child's food. Check the label of any food product you use to make family meals.

- The best way for your child to learn to eat and enjoy new foods is to copy you. Try to eat with them as often as you can.

- Give small portions and praise your child for eating, even if they only eat a little.

- If your child rejects the food, don't force them to eat it. Just take the food away without saying anything. Try to stay calm, even if it's very frustrating. Try the food again another time.

- Don't leave meals until your child is too hungry or tired to eat.

- Your child may be a slow eater, so be patient.

- Don't give your child too many snacks between meals – 2 healthy snacks a day is plenty.

- It's best not to use food as a reward. Your child may start to think of sweets as nice and vegetables as nasty. Instead, reward them with a trip to the park or promise to play a game with them.

- Make mealtimes enjoyable and not just about eating. Sit down and chat about other things.

- If you know any other children of the same age who are good eaters, ask them round for tea. But don't talk too much about how good the other children are.

- Ask an adult that your child likes and looks up to to eat with you. Sometimes a child will eat for someone else, such as a grandparent, without any fuss.

- Changing how you serve a food may make it more appealing. For example, your child might refuse cooked carrots but enjoy raw grated carrot.

NHS Choices
www.nhs.uk

Used by permission.

Appendix 3

What to feed young children

Like the rest of the family, your toddler needs to eat a variety of foods.

Here are some tips on the different sorts of food to offer your child, plus a few it's best to avoid.

Fruit and vegetables

Fruit and vegetables contain lots of vitamins, minerals and fibre. It's good to introduce lots of different types from an early age, whether fresh, frozen, canned or dried, so your baby can enjoy new textures and flavours. Try to make sure fruit and vegetables are included in every meal.

Dried fruit, such as raisins, should be given to your toddler with meals, rather than as a snack in between, as the sugar they contain can cause tooth decay.

Different fruit and vegetables contain different vitamins and minerals, so the more different types your toddler eats, the better.

Don't worry if they'll only eat one or two types at first. Keep offering them small amounts of other fruit and vegetables so they can learn to like different tastes.

Some children don't like cooked vegetables, but will nibble on raw vegetables while you're preparing a meal.

Bread, rice, potatoes, pasta and other starchy foods

Starchy foods, such as bread, breakfast cereals, potatoes, yams, rice, couscous, pasta and chapattis[1] provide energy, nutrients and some fibre.

You can give your child wholegrain foods, such as wholemeal bread, pasta and brown rice. But it's not a good idea to only give wholegrain starchy foods to under-2s.

_____

1 *(In Indian cooking) a thin pancake of unleavened wholemeal bread cooked on a griddle. (Oxford Dictionary)*

Wholegrain foods can be high in fibre and they may fill your child up before they have taken in the calories and nutrients they need. After age 2 you can gradually introduce more wholegrain foods.

Milk and dairy products

Milk

Breast milk is the only food or drink babies need in the first 6 months of their life. It's best to carry on breastfeeding alongside an increasingly varied diet once you introduce solid foods.

Infant formula is the only suitable alternative to breast milk in the first 12 months of your baby's life. Whole cows' milk can be given as a main drink from the age of 1.

Whole milk and full-fat dairy products are a good source of calcium, which helps your child develop strong bones and teeth.

They also contain vitamin A, which helps the body resist infections and is needed for healthy skin and eyes.

Try to give your child at least 350ml (12oz) of milk a day, or 2 servings of foods made from milk, such as cheese, yoghurt or frsomage frais.

Semi-skimmed milk can be introduced from the age of 2, provided your child is a good eater and growing well for their age.

Skimmed or 1% fat milk doesn't contain enough fat, so isn't recommended for children under 5. You can use them in cooking from the age of 1, though.

You can give your child unsweetened calcium-fortified milk alternatives, such as soya, almond and oat drinks, from the age of 1 as part of a healthy, balanced diet.

Toddlers and young children under the age of 5 shouldn't have rice drinks because of the levels of arsenic they contain.

If your child has an allergy or intolerance to milk, talk to your health visitor or GP. They can advise you on suitable milk alternatives.

Cheese

Cheese can form part of a healthy, balanced diet for babies and young children, and provides calcium, protein and vitamins like vitamin A.

Babies can eat pasteurised full-fat cheese from 6 months old. This includes hard cheeses, such as mild cheddar cheese, cottage cheese and cream cheese.

Full-fat cheeses and dairy products are recommended up to the age of 2, as young children need fat and energy to help them grow.

Babies and young children shouldn't eat mould-ripened soft cheeses, such as brie[2] or camembert[3], ripened goats' milk cheese like chèvre[4], and soft blue veined cheese like roquefort[5].

These cheeses may be made from unpasteurised milk and may therefore carry bacteria called listeria.

You can check labels on cheeses to make sure they're made from pasteurised milk.

But these cheeses can be used as part of a cooked recipe as listeria is killed by cooking – baked brie, for example, is a safer option.

Beans, pulses, fish, eggs, meat and other proteins

Young children need protein and iron to grow and develop. Try to give your toddler one or two portions from this group each day.

Beans, pulses, fish, eggs, foods made from pulses (such as tofu, hummus and soya mince) and meat are excellent sources of protein and iron.

Nuts also contain protein, but whole nuts, including peanuts, shouldn't be given to children under 5 in case they choke.

It's recommended that boys have no more than 4 portions of oily fish (such as mackerel, salmon and sardines) a week, and girls no more than 2 portions a week.

This is because oily fish can contain low levels of pollutants that can build up in the body.[6]

Remember, don't stop feeding your child oily fish – the health benefits are greater than the risks, as long as they don't eat more than the recommended amounts.

---

2 *A kind of soft, mild, creamy cheese with a firm white skin. (Oxford Dictionary)*

3 *A kind of rich, soft, creamy cheese with a whitish rind, originally made near Camembert in Normandy. (Oxford Dictionary)*

4 *French cheese made with goat's milk. (Oxford Dictionary)*

5 *A soft blue cheese made from ewes' milk. It is ripened in limestone caves and has a strong flavour. (Oxford Dictionary)*

6 *Read more about how much fish children should eat at https://www.nhs.uk/live-well/eat-well/fish-and-shellfish-nutrition/#much2*

Helping your child get enough iron

Iron is essential for your child's health.

It comes in 2 forms:

*   The iron found in meat and fish, which is easily absorbed by the body
*   Iron from plant foods, which isn't as easy for the body to absorb

If your child doesn't eat meat or fish, they'll get enough iron if you give them plenty of other iron-rich foods, such as fortified breakfast cereals, dark green vegetables, broad beans and lentils.

If young children fill up on milk, it makes it difficult for them to get the calories and nutrients they need from a varied diet.

These children are more likely to lack iron, which can lead to iron-deficiency anaemia. This can affect your child's physical and mental development.

Foods containing fat, sugar and salt

Fat

Young children, especially those under the age of 2, need the energy provided by fat. There are also some vitamins that are only found in fats.

This is why foods like whole milk, yoghurt, cheese and oily fish are so important.

Once your child's 2, you can gradually introduce lower fat dairy products and cut down on fat in other foods – provided your child is a good eater and growing well.

By the time your child is 5 they can eat a healthy low-fat diet like the one recommended for adults.

Keep an eye on the amount of fat (particularly saturated fats) in the food your family eats. Try to keep it to a minimum.

The following tips will help you reduce the amount of fat in your family's meals:

Grill or bake foods instead of frying them.

During cooking, skim the fat off meat dishes such as mince or curry.

Buy leaner cuts of meat and lower fat meat products, such as lower fat sausages and burgers.

Take the skin off poultry.

Reduce the amount of meat you put in stews and casseroles. Make up the difference with lentils, split peas or soaked dried beans.

For children over 2, use lower fat dairy products, such as low-fat spreads and reduced-fat cheeses.

Use as little cooking oil as possible. Choose one that's high in mono- or polyunsaturates, such as rapeseed, soya or olive oil. In the UK, oil labelled vegetable oil is often actually rapeseed oil.

Sugar

Brushing your child's teeth regularly and visits to the dentist are essential to help keep your child's teeth healthy.

It's also important to keep the amount of added sugar they have to a minimum. Added sugar is found in fizzy drinks, juice drinks, sweets, cakes and jam.

It's best to offer your toddler water or whole milk to drink. Semi-skimmed milk can be introduced once they're 2 years old.

You can also offer diluted fruit juice (1 part juice to 10 parts water) served with meals. Serving it with a meal helps to reduce the risk of tooth decay.

From age 5, it's OK to give your child undiluted fruit juice or smoothies, but stick to no more than 1 glass (about 150ml) a day served with a meal.

The sugar in raisins and other dried fruits can cause tooth decay. It's best to give these to your toddler with meals rather than as a snack in between.

Salt

There's no need to add salt to your child's food. Most foods already contain enough salt.

Too much salt can give your child a taste for salty foods and contribute to high blood pressure in later life.

Your whole family will benefit if you gradually reduce the amount of salt in your cooking. Try to limit the amount of salty foods your child has, and always check food labels.

NHS Choices
www.nhs.uk

Used by permission.

Appendix 4

Meal ideas

Baby and toddler meal ideas

If you need some inspiration to help you cook healthy and tasty food for your kids, try these meal ideas.

They're not suitable as first foods, but fine once your baby is used to eating a wide range of solid foods.

When preparing food for babies, don't add salt, sugar or stock cubes directly to the food, or to the cooking water.

Breakfast ideas for babies and children

- Unsweetened porridge or cereal mixed with milk, topped with mashed ripe pear
- Wholewheat biscuit cereal with milk and unsweetened stewed fruit
- Toast fingers with mashed banana
- Toast fingers with a hard-boiled egg and slices of ripe peach
- Unsweetened stewed apple and breakfast cereal with plain, unsweetened yoghurt

Children's lunch or tea ideas

- Cauliflower cheese with cooked pasta pieces
- Mashed pasta with broccoli and cheese
- Baked beans (reduced salt and sugar) with toast
- Scrambled egg with toast, chapatti or pitta bread
- Cottage cheese dip with pitta bread and cucumber and carrot sticks
- Plain fromage frais with stewed apple

Children's dinners

- Mashed sweet potato with mashed chickpeas and cauliflower

- Shepherd's pie (made with beef or lamb) with green vegetables
- Rice and mashed peas with courgette sticks
- Mashed cooked lentils with rice
- Minced chicken and vegetable casserole with mashed potato
- Mashed canned salmon with couscous and peas
- Fish poached in milk with potato, broccoli and carrot

Snacks for babies and toddlers

- Fresh fruit, such as small pieces of soft, ripe peeled pear or peach
- Canned fruit in fruit juice
- Rice pudding or porridge (with no added sugar or salt)
- Plain, unsweetened yoghurt
- Toast, pitta or chapatti fingers
- Unsalted and unsweetened rice cakes
- Plain bagels
- Small cubes of cheese

Getting your child to eat fruit and vegetables

To increase your child's intake of fruit and vegetables, try:

- Putting their favourite vegetables or canned pineapple on top of pizza
- Giving them carrot sticks, slices of pepper and peeled apple as snacks
- Mixing chopped or mashed vegetables with rice, mashed potatoes, meat sauces or dhal[1]
- Chopping prunes or dried apricots into cereal or plain, unsweetened yoghurt, or adding them to a stew
- Mixing fruit (fresh, canned or stewed) with plain, unsweetened yoghurt for a tasty dessert; you could also try tinned fruit

---

1 (In Indian cooking) split pulses, in particular lentils. (Oxford Dictionary)

in fruit juice, such as pears and peaches, or unsweetened stewed fruit, such as apples

Your baby and cows' milk

- From 6 months, keep giving your child breast milk or formula milk, as well as introducing solid foods, but don't give cows' milk as a drink.

- Whole cows' milk can be used in small amounts in cooking or mixed with foods from the age of 6 months. You can give it to your child as a drink from 1 year of age.

- Semi-skimmed milk can be introduced at 2 years old, providing your child is eating a varied diet and growing well for their age. From 5 years, you can give your child 1% or skimmed milk to drink.

NHS Choices
www.nhs.uk

Used by permission.

NHS Choices (www.nhs.uk) was launched in 2007 and is the official website of the National Health Service in England.

We encourage to visit the site of NHS Choices at www.nhs.uk to reach further advice about toddlers and children nutrition and behaviour. The content is available in the chapter "Fussy eaters"[1] and the section "Your pregnancy and baby guide"[2].

----

1 https://www.nhs uk/conditions/pregnancy-and-baby/fussy-eaters/

2 https://www.nhs uk/conditions/pregnancy-and-baby/

Interesting to read

Nutrition Australia.

For Panicky Parents with Fussy Eaters [Online]. Available at: http://www.nutritionaustralia.org/national/resource/panicky-parents-fussy-eaters

References

Addessi, E.; Galloway, A.T.; Visalberghi, E.; Birch, L.L. (2005). Specific social influences on the acceptance of novel foods in 2–5-year-old children. *Appetite*, 45, 264–271

Anon (2018). *Melomakarona - Honey Cookies with Walnuts*. About.com. Available at: http://greekfood.about.com/od/cookiescakes/r/Melomakarona-Spiced-Honey-Cookies-With-Walnuts.htm [Accessed: 6 July 2018]..

BabyCentre UK (2015) *sss* [Online]. Available at: https://www.babycentre.co.uk/x552305/why-is-my-toddler-such-a-fussy-eater [Accessed: 5 July 2018].

Brown, C.L., Perrin, E.M., Peterson, K.E., Brophy Herb, H.E., Horodynski, M.A., Contreras, D., Miller, A.L., et al. (2018). Association of Picky Eating With Weight Status and Dietary Quality Among Low-Income *Preschoolers*. Academic Pediatrics [Online] 18:334–341. Available at: http://www.ncbi.nlm.nih.gov/pubmed/28887030 [Accessed: 3 July 2018].

Chao, H.-C. (2018). Association of Picky Eating with Growth, Nutritional Status, Development, Physical Activity, and Health in Preschool Children. *Frontiers in pediatrics* [Online] 6:22. Available at: http://www.ncbi.nlm.nih.gov/pubmed/29484290 [Accessed: 3 July 2018].

Fernandez, C., DeJesus, J.M., Miller, A.L., Appugliese, D.P., Rosenblum, K.L., Lumeng, J.C. and Pesch, M.H. (2018). Selective eating behaviors in children: An observational validation of parental report measures. *Appetite* [Online] 127:163–170. Available at: http://www.ncbi.nlm.nih.gov/pubmed/29729326 [Accessed: 3 July 2018].

Harris Interactive (2018). Which of the Following People, If Any, Do You Consider to Be Picky Eaters? [Online]. Available at: https://www.statista.com/statistics/426021/picky-eaters-in-the-united-states/ [Accessed: 3 July 2018].

Koivisto, U.K.; Sjoden, P.G. (1996). Reasons for rejection of food items in Swedish families with children aged 2–17. *Appetite* 1996, 26, 89–103.

Kwon, K., Shim, J., Kang, M. and Paik, H.-Y. (2017). Association between Picky Eating Behaviors and Nutritional Status in Early Childhood: Performance of a Picky Eating Behavior Questionnaire. *Nutrients* [Online] 9:463. Available at: http://www.mdpi.com/2072-6643/9/5/463.

Maranhão, H. de S., Aguiar, R.C. de, Lira, D.T.J. de, Sales, M.Ú.F. and Nóbrega, N.Á. do N. (2018). Feeding Difficulties in Preschool Children, Previous Feeding Practices, and Nutritional Status. Revista paulista de pediatria : *orgao oficial da Sociedade de Pediatria de Sao Paulo* [Online] 36:7. Available at: http://www.ncbi.nlm.nih.gov/pubmed/29091129 [Accessed: 3 July 2018].

Mascola, A.J., Bryson, S.W and Agras, W.S. (2010). Picky eating during childhood: a longitudinal study to age 11 years. *Eating behaviors* [Online] 11:253–7. Available at: http://www.ncbi.nlm.nih.gov/pubmed/20850060 [Accessed: 3 July 2018].

Nansel, T.R., Lipsky, L.M., Haynie, D.L., Eisenberg, M.H., Dempster, K. and Liu, A. (2018). Picky Eaters Improved Diet Quality in a Randomized Behavioral Intervention Trial in Youth with Type 1 Diabetes. *Journal of the Academy of Nutrition and Dietetics* [Online] 118:308–316. Available at: http://www.ncbi.nlm.nih.gov/pubmed/29389510 [Accessed: 3 July 2018].

NHS.UK. *Fussy Eaters*, NHS Choices [Online]. Available at: https://www.nhs.uk/conditions/pregnancy-and-baby/fussy-eaters

NHS.UK. *Dealing with child behaviour problems*, NHS Choices [Online]. Available at: https://www.nhs.uk/conditions/pregnancy-and-baby/dealing-with-difficult-behaviour/

NHS.UK. *What to feed young children*, NHS Choices [Online]. Available at: https://www.nhs.uk/conditions/pregnancy-and-baby/understanding-food-groups/

NHS.UK. *Meal ideas*, NHS Choices [Online]. Available at: https://www.nhs.uk/conditions/pregnancy-and-baby/childrens-meal-ideas/

Nutrition Australia. *For Panicky Parents with Fussy Eaters* [Online]. Available at: http://www.nutrition-australia.org/national/resource/panicky-parents-fussy-eaters [Accessed: 3 July 2018].

Oxford University Press (2018). *Oxford Dictionaries* [Online]. Available at: https://en.oxforddictionaries.com/ [Accessed: 22 June 2018].

Podlesak, A.K., Mozer, M.E., Smith-Simpson, S., Lee, S.-Y. and Donovan, S.M. (2017). Associations between Parenting Style and Parent and Toddler Mealtime Behaviors. *Current developments in nutrition* [Online] 1:e000570. Available at: http://www.ncbi.nlm.nih.gov/pubmed/29955704 [Accessed: 3 July 2018].

Sakkas, P. (2015). *Revealing Psychiatry... from an Insider*. London: Stergiou Limited.

Taylor, C.M., Wernimont, S.M., Northstone, K. and Emmett, P.M. (2015). Picky/fussy eating in children: Review of definitions, assessment, prevalence and dietary intakes. *Appetite* [Online] 95:349–359. Available at: https://www.sciencedirect.com/science/article/pii/S0195666315003438 [Accessed: 3 July 2018].

Bibliography

Allen, K.L., Byrne, S.M. and Crosby, R.D. (2015). Distinguishing Between Risk Factors for Bulimia Nervosa, Binge Eating Disorder, and Purging Disorder. *Journal of Youth and Adolescence* 44:1580–1591.

Altinyazar, V. and Maner, F. (2014). Eating disorders and psychosis. *Anatolian Journal of Psychiatry*

American Psychiatric Association (APA) (2013). Feeding and Eating Disorders Fact Sheet. *Diagnostic and Statistical Manual of Mental Disorders (DSM-5)*:1–2.

B.M., P. and S.R., W. (2002). Interventions for preventing eating disorders in children and adolescents. *Cochrane* Allen, K.L., Byrne, S.M. and Crosby, R.D. (2015). Distinguishing Between Risk Factors for Bulimia Nervosa, Binge Eating Disorder, and Purging Disorder. *Journal of Youth and Adolescence* 44:1580–1591.

Altinyazar, V. and Maner, F. (2014). Eating disorders and psychosis. *Anatolian Journal of Psychiatry*

American Psychiatric Association (APA) (2013). Feeding and Eating Disorders Fact Sheet. *Diagnostic and Statistical Manual of Mental Disorders (DSM-5)*:1–2.

B.M., P. and S.R., W. (2002). Interventions for preventing eating disorders in children and adolescents. *Cochrane database of systematic reviews*

Barton, R. and Nicholls, D. (2008). Management of eating disorders in children and adolescents. *Psychiatry* 7:167–170.

Başkale, H. and Bahar, Z. (2011). Outcomes of nutrition knowledge and healthy food choices in 5- to 6-year-old children who received a nutrition intervention based on Piaget's theory. *Journal for Specialists in Pediatric Nursing* 16:263–279.

Blissett, J. and Haycraft, E. (2011). Parental eating disorder symptoms and observations of mealtime interactions with children. *Journal of Psychosomatic Research* 70:368–371.

Blodgett Salafia, E.H., Jones, M.E., Haugen, E.C. and Schaefer, M.K. (2015). Perceptions of the causes of eating disorders: A comparison of individuals with and without eating disorders. *Journal of Eating Disorders* 3.

Bravender, T., Bryant-Waugh, R., Herzog, D., Katzman, D., Kriepe, R.D., Lask, B., Le Grange, D., *et al.* (2010). Classification of eating disturbance in children and adolescents: Proposed changes for the DSM-V. *European Eating Disorders Review* 18:79–89.

Bryant-Waugh, R. and Watkins, B. (2015). Feeding and eating disorders. In: *Rutter's Child and Adolescent Psychiatry: Sixth Edition.* pp. 1016–1034.

Bydlowski, S., Corcos, M., Jeammet, P., Paterniti, S., Berthoz, S., Laurier, C., Chambry, J., *et al.* (2005). Emotion-processing deficits in eating disorders. *International Journal of Eating Disorders* 37:321–329.

Campbell, K. and Peebles, R. (2014). Eating Disorders in Children and Adolescents: State of the Art Review. *PEDIATRICS*

Cassin, S.E. and Von Ranson, K.M. (2005). Personality and eating disorders: A decade in review. *Clinical Psychology Review* 25:895–916.

Chatoor, I. and Khushlani, D. (2006). Eating disorders. In: *Handbook of Preschool Mental Health: Development, Disorders, and Treatment.* pp. 115–136.

Cimino, S., Cerniglia, L. and Paciello, M. (2015). Mothers with Depression, Anxiety or Eating Disorders: Outcomes on Their Children and the Role of Paternal Psychological Profiles. *Child Psychiatry and Human Development* 46:228–236.

Couturier, J. and Rutherford, L. (2007). A Review of Psychotherapeutic Interventions for children and adolescents with eating disorders. *Journal of the Canadian Academy of Child and Adolescent Psychiatry*

Cruchet, S., Lucero, Y. and Cornejo, V. (2016). Truths, Myths and Needs of Special Diets: Attention-Deficit/Hyperactivity Disorder, Autism, Non-Celiac Gluten Sensitivity, and Vegetarianism. *Annals of Nutrition and Metabolism* 68:43–50.

Dovey, T.M., Staples, P.A., Gibson, E.L. and Halford, J.C.G. (2008). Food neophobia and 'picky/fussy' eating in children: A review. *Appetite* 50:181–193.

Eddy, K.T., Le Grange, D., Crosby, R.D., Hoste, R.R., Doyle, A.C., Smyth, A. and Herzog, D.B. (2010). Diagnostic Classification of Eating Disorders in Children and Adolescents: How Does DSM-IV-TR Compare to Empirically-Derived Categories? *Journal of the American Academy of Child and Adolescent Psychiatry* 49:277–287.

Eddy, K.T., Novotny, C.M. and Westen, D. (2004). Sexuality, personality, and eating disorders. *Eating Disorders* 12:191–208.

El-Radhi, A.S. (2015). Appropriate care for children with eating disorders and obesity. *British Journal of Nursing* [Online] 24:518–522.

Elran-Barak, R., Sztainer, M., Goldschmidt, A.B. and Le Grange, D. (2014). Family meal frequency among children and adolescents with eating disorders. *Journal of Adolescent Health* 55:53–58.

Equit, M., Pälmke, M., Becker, N., Moritz, A.-M., Becker, S. and von Gontard, A. (2013). Eating problems in young children -- a population-based study. *Acta paediatrica (Oslo, Norway : 1992)*

Fitzpatrick, K.K., Lesser, J., Brandenburg, B. and Lesser, J. (2011). Addressing low self-esteem in adolescents with eating disorders. *Adolescent Psychiatry*

Forsberg, S. and Lock, J. (2015). Family-based Treatment of Child and Adolescent Eating Disorders. *Child and Adolescent Psychiatric Clinics of North America* 24:617–629.

Friederich, H.C., Wu, M., Simon, J.J. and Herzog, W. (2013). Neurocircuit function in eating disorders. *International Journal of Eating Disorders* 46:425–432.

Goodier, G.H.G., McCormack, J., Egan, S.J., Watson, H.J., Hoiles, K.J., Todd, G. and Treasure, J.L. (2014). Parent skills training treatment for parents of children and adolescents with eating disorders: A qualitative study. *International Journal of Eating Disorders*

Grange, D. le and Loeb, K.L. (2007). Early identification and treatment of eating disorders: prodrome to syndrome. *Early Intervention in Psychiatry*

Hall, H. (2014). Food Myths. Skeptic [Online] 19:10–19.

Harrison, A., Sullivan, S., Tchanturia, K. and Treasure, J. (2010). Emotional functioning in eating disorders: Attentional bias, emotion recognition and emotion regulation. *Psychological Medicine* 40:1887–1897.

Hudson, L.D. and Court, A.J. (2012). What paediatricians should know about eating disorders in children and young people. *Journal of Paediatrics and Child Health* 48:869–875.

Kass, A.E., Kolko, R.P. and Wilfley, D.E. (2013). Psychological treatments for eating disorders. *Current Opinion in Psychiatry* 26:549–555.

Kennedy, E. (1996). Healthy meals, healthy food choices, healthy children: USDA's team nutrition. In: *Preventive Medicine*. pp. 56–60.

Knez, R., Munjas, R., Petrovečki, M., Paučić-Kirinčić, E. and Peršić, M. (2006). Disordered eating attitudes among elementary school population. *Journal of Adolescent Health* 38:628–630.

Lesser, L.I., Mazza, M.C. and Lucan, S.C. (2015). Nutrition myths and healthy dietary advice in clinical practice. American Family Physician 91:634–638.

Mairs, R. and Nicholls, D. (2016). Assessment and treatment of eating disorders in children and adolescents. *Archives of Disease in Childhood* 101:1168–1175.

Mayo Clinic Staff (2013). Nutrition and healthy eating. *Mayo Clinic*

Nadon, G., Feldman, D.E., Dunn, W. and Gisel, E. (2011). Association of Sensory Processing and Eating Problems in Children with Autism Spectrum Disorders. *Autism Research and Treatment*

Ogata, B.N. and Hayes, D. (2014). Position of the academy of nutrition and dietetics: Nutrition guidance for healthy children ages 2 to 11 years. *Journal of the Academy of Nutrition and Dietetics* 114:1257–1276.

Oxford University Press (2018). Oxford Dictionaries [Online]. Available at: https://en.oxforddictionaries.com

Ricca, V., Rotella, F., Mannucci, E., Ravaldi, C., Castellini, G., Lapi, F., Cangioli, L., *et al.* (2010). Eating behaviour and body satisfaction in mediterranean children: the role of the parents. *Clinical practice and epidemiology in mental health : CP & EMH* 6:59–65.

Sierksma, A. and Kok, F.J. (2012). Beer and health: From myths to science. European Journal of Clinical Nutrition 66:869–870.

Vinci, D.M. (2005). Nutrition Myth Busters. Athletic Therapy Today [Online] 10:48–49.

Index

C

D

L

LDL xv, 16
Leak 37
Leave 37, 93, 114, 133, 134, 136
Lemon vii, 19, 77, 79, 85
Lemon juice 19, 51, 61, 71, 73, 75, 79
Lemon zest 20, 79, 83
Lentil 93
Leonidas Stergiou iv, 150. See also Stergiou, Leonidas
Lice 16
Liquid gold 16
Love 123
Lungs 17
Lycopene 18

M

Magnesium 17, 18, 19
Margarine 47, 53
Raisins 47, 53
Meal vii, viii, x, 30, 32, 36, 38, 42, 44, 46, 48, 50, 58, 62, 66, 68, 70, 72, 74, 78, 80, 82, 106, 135, 139, 150
Meal ideas 1, 135
Meat vii, viii, 21, 43, 45, 47, 59, 63, 67, 69, 73, 75, 91, 94, 96, 97, 102, 112, 113, 114, 115, 117, 123, 128, 132, 133, 134, 136, 147, 150
Meatballs viii, 31, 75, 113
Milk 22, 45, 92, 115, 123
Mint 39, 41, 53, 37, 113, 99
Memories 94
Minced meat viii, 43, 45, 47, 59, 63, 67, 73, 75, 97, 102
Minerals 19, 130
Moderation 19
Motivation 121
Moussaka viii, 95
Moustakas, George iii, iv, vi, x, xiii, 1, 96, 156, 157
Mushrooms 123

N

National Health Service. See also NHS.UK Choices; NHS.UK; NHS Choices; www.NHS.Uk
Natural protein 18
Neophobia 8, 124, 143
Neophobic behaviour 124
Nervous system 15
NHS choices 14, 106, 127, 129, 134, 137, 139
NHS.Uk 127, 129, 132, 134, 137, 139
NHS.Uk choices iv, 12, 15
Nutrition 1, 7, 132, 137, 140, 141, 144, 145

O

P

R

Stergiou Limited
International edition

EAN 13: 0616316146006
SKU: 9781912315369

ISBN
978-1-912315-36-9 (print, paperback, primary)
978-1-912315-18-5 (print, paperback, Amazon edition)
978-1-912315-19-2 (eBook, standard/reflowable)
978-1-912315-35-2 (eBook, fixed-layout/print replica)

Imprint
Stergiou Limited

Subject Codes
CKB119000: COOKING / Cooking for Kids
PSY011000: Psychology : Psychopathology - Eating Disorders
CKB120000: COOKING / Cooking with Kids

Thema
MKZD - Eating disorders & therapy
WBQ - Cooking for/with children

Audience
Trade/General (Adult)

Book Type
Standard Colour 5.5 x 8.5 in or 216 x 140 mm (Demy 8vo)
Perfect Bound on Standard 70 White w/Gloss Lam
Page Count: 176
Spine Width: 0.478 in
Weight: 0.623 lbs

Printer and distribution network
Australia, Brazil, Canada, China, European Union(Germany, Italy, Poland,
Spain, United Kingdom), India, Russia, South Korea, United States.

Global distributors
 Stergiou Limited, Ingram

The Authors

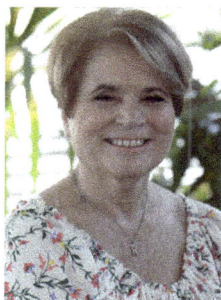

EIRINI TOGIA

. . . .

By the same author

. . . .

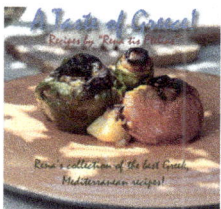

Paperback
ISBN: 9781910370551
Hardcover
ISBN: 9781910370537
eBook
ISBN: 9781910370056

Pages: 100
Language: English

Greek edition
Paperback
ISBN: 9781910370544
Hardcover
ISBN: 9781910370292
eBook
ISBN: 9781910370094

Eirini Togia, well-known as "Rena tis Ftelias", was born in Corfu and lives in Athens. She started her first restaurant in Mykonos at the Ftelia beach in 1979, and soon, the restaurant became a must-visit place for Greek and international celebrities and those appreciative of good-quality food. Six years later, she opened a boutique restaurant in Athens. For several years, both restaurants operated simultaneously.

Rena has been a true representative of the Greek Mediterranean cuisine for over 39 years now and is very well-known for her hospitality and her respect and love for pure, fresh ingredients (virgin olive oil, vegetables and herbs). Her recipes are simple and authentic, and they reflect the Greek tradition and culture. For several consecutive years, Rena's restaurant has been distinguished and shortlisted amongst the top restaurants in Athens with individual and corporate customers from Greece and abroad.

Rena has published several cookbooks in Greek and other languages that have received numerous European and international distinctions.

Two of her books, namely *Greek Mediterranean Cuisine* and *Rena's Desserts*, received a distinction in the International Gourmand Cookbook Contest in 2004 in Barcelona, and Rena was awarded the "2nd Best Woman Chef in the World".

In 2008, Rena represented Greece in the "Greek Gastronomy Week" held by the Greek National Tourism Organization in China and participated in the "International Tourism Exhibition", organised again by the Greek National Tourism Organization.

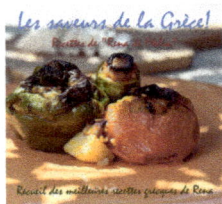

Paperback
ISBN: 9781910370582
Hardcover
ISBN: 9781910370605
eBook
ISBN: 978-1-910370-59-9
Pages: 100
Language: French

In 2015, she gained two Gourmand World Awards —"Best Woman Chef Book - Best in the World" and "Best Translation Book in Greece"— for the English and French editions of her book *A Taste of Greece* (original Greek title *Ρένα της Φτελιάς: Συνταγές που Αγαπήσαμε*), respectively (published by Stergiou Limited). In 2016, these titles were finalists in China's event for the "Wine and Drinks books" and "Cookbooks and Food Culture" categories.

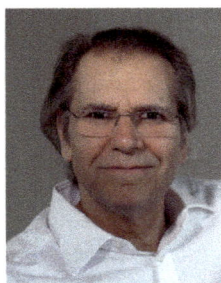

PAVLOS SAKKAS

By the same author

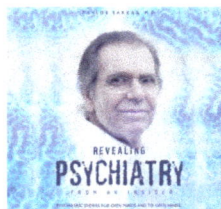

Audiobook
ASIN: B018T4LTQ2

Length: 11h 48m
Language: English

Pavlos Sakkas grew up in the milieu of psychiatry as his father was also a psychiatrist. Pavlos has practised psychiatry on the front lines for the last thirty years and is a Professor of Psychiatry at the Medical School of the University of Athens. He has also been a Visiting Professor at the University of Illinois in Chicago. He has obtained prestigious scholarships and has accomplished substantial works in research, with hundreds of publications in international scientific journals.

However, despite these great professional achievements, his greatest fondness is for teaching. He has spent his long academic career initiating thousands of medical students and hundreds of specialised psychiatrists into the world of psychiatry. Furthermore, featured in the media on numerous occasions, he tries to familiarise the general public with the messages of modern psychiatry and the significant developments achieved in recent decades.

Pavlos Sakkas' inquisitive spirit has formulated fresh and enterprising points of view concerning certain aspects – that are still obscure – of psychiatry. In his clinical work, which has been met with high esteem, he has, meanwhile, applied special personal techniques of approach to a patient. It is these views and employed techniques that are set out in his present book, which represents the distillation of his knowledge and experience.

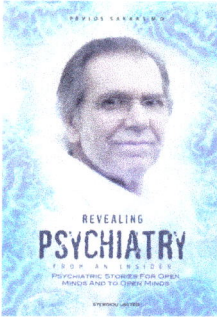

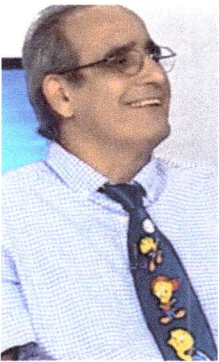

Paperback
ISBN: 9781910370735
eBook
ISBN: 9781910370742

Pages: 252
Language: English

The paediatrician George Moustakas studied at the Medical School of the National and Kapodistrian University of Athens. He received a speciality in paediatrics title at the tier 1 University Paediatric Clinic of Children's Hospital in Greece, "Aglaia Kyriakou".

He was a volunteer at the Olympic Games in Athens in 2004 and the Special Olympics in 2011. George took active voluntary actions on paediatric prophylactic control in various humanitarian childhood institutions such as "Children's Smile" and many more.

GEORGE MOUSTAKAS

During his many years as a paediatrician, George has been involved in various humanitarian missions during wars and natural disasters in different places of the world (Yugoslavia, Kosovo, etc.).

He has participated in various medical publications with paediatric issues such as diet, vaccination, accidents, and tips on ther as well as in international specialised paediatric congresses such as those in the

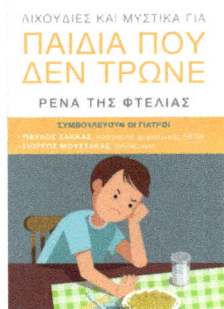

ΛΙΧΟΥΔΙΕΣ ΚΑΙ ΜΥΣΤΙΚΑ ΓΙΑ
ΠΑΙΔΙΑ ΠΟΥ
ΔΕΝ ΤΡΩΝΕ

ΡΕΝΑ ΤΗΣ ΦΤΕΛΙΑΣ

By Eirini Togia,
Pavlos Sakkas
George Moustakas

Paperback
ISBN: 9781912315161
eBook
ISBN: 9781912315178

Pages: 152
Language: Greek

USA (Chicago, San Francisco, Texas), in Europe (UK, France, Germany, Sweden, Ireland, Portugal etc.), China, Thailand, Hong Kong, Beijing, and hundreds of paediatric congresses in Greece.

He has been practising paediatrics at the Athens Paediatric Centre since 1992 and in the paediatric department of the Journalists' Fund (EDOEAP) the past 20 years until today. He is a member of the Athens Medical Association and the Greek Paediatric Society.

The translator and copy-editor

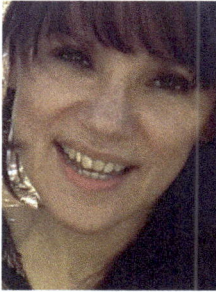

CATHERINE PAVLOU EVANS

Catherine Pavlou Evans was born in Athens, Greece in 1960. She studied public and European law at the University of Lille in France and obtained her Master's degree from the University of Perpignan (France). Her career covers a wide range of occupations – and a long span of time – from office clerk to general manager and HR director, from probate lawyer to the position of assistant professor of constitutional and public law. She has travelled quite a lot, and she lives in Greece where she teaches Greek, French, and English. She translates from Greek, English, French, and Italian to Greek and English.

Catherine has written a compilation about *Famous Greek Women*. She used to write for *Serendipity Magazine Online*. She is the author of In the *Beginning, There Was X*, a social science fiction book published in 2006 by Arima Publishing in the UK. The book is available on Amazon and arimapublishing. com. She also wrote the Greek novel *Ένα σύμπαν μιλφέιγ* (In English, *A Millefeuille Universe*), which was published in 2015 by Fereniki Publications in Greece.

Currently, she is writing her new book, co-authoring a script for a thriller, and hoping to find the time – and the discipline – to translate her "X" book into Greek. She is also a radio producer.

You may contact her at catpavlou@gmail. com and on her Facebook profile, "Catherine Pavlou". Both of her books have their own Facebook pages, each under the book's title.

Also published by Stergiou Limited

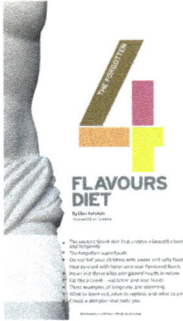

The Forgotten Four Flavours Diet
By Elias Kefalidis

The Four Flavours is a diet that promotes longevity, helps to lose weight, and improves health. This book describes a holistic nutritional system that evolved from ancient Greece, and has attracted worldwide medical interest.

Paperback ISBN: 978-1-910370-75-9
eBook ISBN: 978-1-910370-76-6

Pages: 120
Language: English

www.ingramcontent.com/pod-product-compliance
Lightning Source LLC
Chambersburg PA
CBHW041220030426
42336CB00024B/3401